Needs to know: a guide to needs assessment for primary care

To Genevieve, Eloise and Constance

A Need to know:

There is a need, bitter need, to bring back, if we may, into men's minds, that to live is nothing unless to live be known by Him by whom we live, and that is not to be known amidst the hurry of crowds and crash of innovation, but in solitary places, and out of the glowing intelligence which He gave to men of old

Ruskin

Synopsis of editor

Andrew Harris is a Senior Registrar in Public Health in City and East London Health Authority. He has spent 11 years in general practice and has an honorary academic post at King's College Hospital Medical School, London, continuing some teaching and training. He has been an FHSA director for 3 years, with responsibilities for health strategies, before retraining in public health medicine. His attachment to Tower Hamlets Health Care Trust enabled him to conduct needs assessments of the young physically disabled population. His publications cover a wide area – health policy, violence in general practice, screening public health roles and primary care evaluation. His current interest is the primary care/public health interface in a primary care-led NHS.

For Churchill Livingstone

Commissioning Editor: Peter Richardson
Project Editor: Prudence Daniels
Project Controller: Mark Sanderson

Freelance

Copy Editor: Rich Cutler
Proof Reader: Ian Ross
Indexer: Katie Izat
Cover Design: Andrew Jones

Needs to know:
a guide to needs assessment for primary care

Edited by

Andrew Harris

Senior Registrar in Public Health,
East London & City Health Authority,
Honorary Lecturer in General Practice,
King's College Hospital Medical & Dental School,
London, UK

CHURCHILL LIVINGSTONE
NEW YORK EDINBURGH LONDON MADRID MELBOURNE SAN FRANCISCO TOKYO 1997

CHURCHILL LIVINGSTONE
Medical Division of Pearson Professional
Limited

Distributed in the United States of America by Churchill
Livingstone Inc., 650 Avenue of the Americas, New York,
N.Y. 10011, and by associated companies, branches and
representatives throughout the world.

First published 1997

ISBN 0-443-0-05569-6

British Library Cataloguing in Publication Data
A catalogue record for this book is available from the British
Library.

Library of Congress Cataloging in Publication Data
A catalog record for this book is available from the Library of
Congress.

Medical knowledge is constantly changing. As new
information becomes available, changes in treatment,
procedures, equipment and the use of drugs become
necessary. The editors, authors, contributors and the
publishers have, as far as possible, taken care to ensure that
the information given in this text is accurate and up to date.
However, readers are strongly advised to confirm that the
information, especially with regard to drug usage, complies
with the latest legislation and standards of practice.

Printed by Bell and Bain Ltd., Glasgow

Contents

Contributors

David Black DipEd, Dip Health Ed, MSc
Freelance Public Health Consultant,
Communicable Health,
Glasgow, UK

Andrew Brooke MB, ChB, DRCOG, MRCGP
General Practitioner,
Gloucester, UK

Valerie Chisty
Consultant in Public Health Medicine,
NHS Executive West Midlands,
Birmingham, UK

Pauline Craig BSc(Hons), RGN, HV
Freelance Public Health Consultant,
Communicable Health,
Glasgow, UK

Yvonne Doyle MB, MRCPI, MSPHM, FSPHMI, MPH, DCH
Senior Lecturer in Public Health,
South East Institute of Public Health,
Tunbridge Wells,
Kent, UK

Nigel Edwards
Director,
London Health Economics Consortium,
London, UK

John Gabbay MB, ChB, MSc, FFPHM
Professor of Public Health Medicine and Director,
Wessex Institute of Public Health Medicine,
University of Southampton,
Southampton, UK

Mark Gabbay MB, ChB, MRCGP, Dip Psychotherapy
Clinical Lecturer in General Practice,
University of Manchester,
Manchester, UK

Stephen Gillam MRCP, MRCGP, MFPHM
Consultant in Public Health Medicine/Primary Care,
Bedfordshire, UK

Liz Haggard
Fellow in Organizational Development,
Office for Public Management,
London, UK

Andrew Harris MB, BChir, MRCP, MSc
Senior Registrar in Public Health,
East London and City Health Authority;
Honorary Lecturer in General Practice,
King's College Hospital Medical and Dental School,
London, UK

Judith Hooper MRCGP, DRCOG, MSc, MFPHM
Consultant in Public Health Medicine,
Calderdale and Kirklees Health Authority,
Huddersfield, UK

Jane Hopton
Research Psychologist,
Department of General Practice,
University of Edinburgh,
Edinburgh, UK

Sadru Kheraj
General Practitioner,
Yeagh House Surgery,
Loughborough Road,
London, UK

George Leahy
Health Economist,
East London & City Health Authority,
London, UK

Tom Marshall MB, ChB, MSc(Health Econ.), MRCGP, MSc(Public Health)
Specialist Registrar in Public Health Medicine,
Northamptonshire Health Authority,
Northampton, UK

Scott A. Murray MD, MRCGP, DCH, DRCOG
Senior Lecturer,
Department of General Practice,
Edinburgh University,
Edinburgh, UK

Chrissie Pickin MB, ChB, MSc, MFPHM
Director of Public Health,
Salford and Trafford Health Authority,
Manchester, UK

Mike Sadler MFPHM, MRCGP, MSc
Consultant in Public Health Medicine,
Portsmouth and South East Hampshire Health
Commission,
Portsmouth, UK

John Shanks
Consultant in Public Health Medicine,
Lambeth, Southwark and Lewisham Health Commission,
London, UK

Andrew Stevens MB, BS, MSc, FFCM
Senior Lecturer in Public Health,
Wessex Institute of Public Health Medicine,
University of Southampton,
Southampton, UK

Sarah Ann Ujah MSc, BSc
Management Consultant,
Bermuda Hospitals Board,
MOH,
Hamilton, Bermuda

Ian Williamson BA(Hons), DipHSM, MPH
Development Manager,
Sefton Health Authority,
Merseyside, UK

Laurann Yen BSc, MPsych
Director of Primary Care and Development Services,
Tower Hamlets Healthcare Trust,
London, UK

Preface

This book was born partly from the confusion and professional dissonance about what is needs assessment. I overheard a comment by a Director of Public Health to the effect that the best needs assessments are done in department corridors. This suggested that there could be a way of bringing disparate professional and managerial views together, perhaps dispensing with the conventional views of each. This book is essentially pragmatic, bringing together both the experience of those in the field, and asking the question 'what impact did the assessment have on practice, attitudes and decision making?' There is no magic answer. Every reader must judge for themselves whether the techniques or practice described make the process of making value judgements about health care any easier, or clinical practice any more effective.

It has been made possible by the generosity and commitment of many in health authorities, and departments of general practice who responded to a national survey of needs assessment activity in primary care. A combination of intelligence from the literature and the field has been put together, as far as possible, linking theory and practice. Primary care assessment is a new field and some contributors have been unable to find examples of some approaches being used in general practice. But where work has been found, effort has been made to ascertain its process and impact, to enable readers to learn from others' experience.

In selecting case studies and in constructing the book as a whole, a broad approach has been taken to needs assessment. I view this as essential, as it should be common ground for all involved in promoting health, and not a purist doctrine owned by one discipline. My working definition of needs assessment has been

'A systematic investigation into the health of some population, or group of people, sharing a common characteristic, in relation to existing public services, in order to meet a specific enquiry; and using methods which produce a sufficiently robust result, to be capable of influencing policy or practice, promoting the health of that group.'

Contributors have been most accommodating and flexible in collaborating with the editor in ensuring this broad approach is reflected in editing the chapters so that they fit together as a coherent whole. Not all will feel entirely comfortable with my definition but all recognize the value of engaging general practitioners, public health specialists and managers in this joint venture.

Its focus is primary care. This is timely as we are all exploring the nature of a primary care led NHS and the opportunities created by the new White Paper (*Choice and Opportunity – Primary Care: The Future*), which will become law in 1997. It is crucial that needs assessment is applied to primary health care, where decisions about commissioning as well as providing care are increasingly being made. The involvement of general practitioners is essential for another reason. They are pivotal in the health service, witnessing in their everyday professional practice, the lives of countless patients and experiencing their demands. At the heart of needs assessment are judgements about people's needs and demands. GPs are in the privileged position of having an understanding of the scientific approach and the human condition. Their honed skills in managing demand are valuable in constructing needs assessment which aid that task.

The adoption of a broad approach to needs assessment and the embracing of primary and community care has enabled the rich synthesis of art and science, which is primary care needs assessment. The process of primary care needs assessment can be likened to my two year old's birthday present. Constance had a wooden train set of many parts. The five trucks could have been connected empty, and the process go ahead, but that did not tell us very much. That is like collecting disparate raw data. It could consist of less trucks, but at what stage does it no longer become a train? One measure of health may not constitute a needs assessment on its own. If the purpose is to carry people, one carriage may render the service not worth doing; if the carriage with the guard is missing, will it go at all? Some information is key. If all the trucks are there, but they are not connected, it certainly will not go. That would be like trying to do a needs assessment without interrelating the information and data collected. Then Constance could choose what to put on each truck, which amounted to some six or so pieces of different colours and shapes, which could go in more than one combination on the poles on each truck, but some combinations were pretty funny looking and some were impossible. It depended what you wanted the train to do, and to look alike. In other words, each train is different: the constituents of a needs assessment process can vary substantially, and it is an art and science to create one fit for each purpose. I hope Constance has helped demystify the process, and encouraged readers to mix scientific method and creativity.

This book aims to generate interest in the values of health needs assessment, and in doing so stimulate its readers also to assess their own professional needs, together with those of their colleagues. Its impact should be measured not only by its effect on services, but also on the way of achieving fulfilling professional lives, developing skills to change both our professional practice and our immediate environment. Ultimately we all share the goal of promoting the health of our population, and it is timely that we should share the means we are currently using to achieve that goal.

People – colleagues and patients alike – are realists. They know that highlighting unmet need will not itself generate new services. But GPs are only too well aware of the benefits to individuals of sharing problems. Sometimes we will discover that we are striving to meet a need that is less pressing than another that someone else is experiencing. Exchanging these perceptions is clarifying and may be invigorating!

Whatever our professional and public accountability, there is that indefinable personal accountability, that gives us our pride and sense of direction. If this book merely creates a new dimension of work for which to be accountable, it will have failed; if it makes its reader consider how to respond to a demand in the knowledge of different unexpressed needs of others it will have been worthwhile.

There is a gap between what we ask for and what we really need. There is a gap between what we do and what we should do. It is a professional and managerial challenge to know these gaps. Sometimes they are expressed by the loudest shouting lobbyist, whose case may be exaggerated. Other times it is not expressed at all, as the sufferer has neither the skills nor inclination to speak up. 'Needs to know' explores how to find those gaps by providing GPs, managers and public health practitioners with what they need to know.

Andrew Harris
London, September 1996

Acknowledgements

I should like to thank Genevieve and Eloise for permitting me to work at home; and Constance who, in preventing me from doing so in her presence, refrained from scribbling on the copy. The incomprehensibility of my scribbles and edits is compensated by a very gifted range of authors, whose research and commitment have produced some illuminating writing. I am indebted to countless correspondents, who replied to my survey of academic departments and health authorities. In particular, I am grateful to those whose work was crafted into case studies, and to Carlos Sampson, who provided the administrative expertise. I acknowledge the support and encouragement of Diane Plamping, Gerry Bennett, Louise Parsons, Bobbie Jacobson and John Cohen. I admire the trust and vision of Peter Richardson, the patience of Mark Sanderson and the industry of Pru Daniels. This team at Churchill Livingstone in a most friendly and efficient manner, meticulously converted chaotic copy into this book. The editors, contributors and the publishers have, as far as possible, taken care to ensure that the information given in this text is accurate and up to date. However, readers are strongly advised to confirm that the information complies with the latest legislation and standards of practice.

For reasons of style, the male pronoun has been used throughout this book. Therefore references to 'he' and 'his' should equally be taken to include 'she' and 'hers'.

Understanding and planning

1

The language of needs assessment

Andrew Harris   Tom Marshall

Eloise, who is 5 years old, has a favourite refrain, which is, 'I *need* a hug'. Her family learnt from her younger years that failure to respond to this statement results in a drama which inevitably captures our attention. Her sister Genevieve prefers the phrase 'I *want* a hug', and she can be more easily persuaded that she wants something else. Failure to respond, at worst, leads to a quiet withdrawal of cooperation. Parents reading this may reflect that the sisters have different personalities and ages. This undoubtedly is true, but does the difference in behaviour tell us anything about differences between want and need? Is a need a strongly felt want which must be met in order to achieve fulfilment – in the same way that a disadvantage arising from a disability prevents us from carrying out an expected role? Or is a need a want which has been validated, in this example by parental approval or acquiescence? Perhaps Genevieve's desire for a hug in some way does not amount to a need. Perhaps the need is met without asking at other times. Is the everyday usage of these terms helpful to our understanding of their technical meaning in professional usage?

A group of people who were taking part in an activity which required their constant attention were asked if they became aware of their filling bladder during this activity and whether they would describe the emergent feeling as a want or a need to go to the lavatory. Opinion was divided. Some continued the activity even though they felt distracted by the need to empty their bladder. Others felt the need to pass water was stronger than the desire to continue with the task. So here is a lesson for health care: in some circumstances we may regulate certain needs to a lower priority. That is, we appear not to want what we need. This is expressed in Maslow's hierarchy of needs (Fig. 1); those things we need most we may desire least. It also serves to illustrate a concept familiar to economists: that wants are 'relative', and we measure our relative wants against one another. Our behaviour illustrates which of these wants we have accorded highest priority.

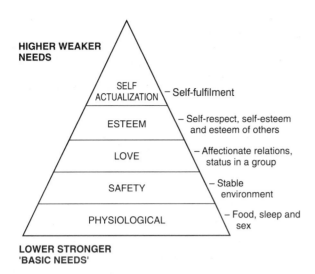

Figure 1.1 Maslow's hierarchy of needs (Cole 1993). A development of the basic model places cognitive needs (to tackle the unknown) and aesthetic needs as two additional ones on the peak of the pyramid.

According to Maslow, in general, needs for sustenance must be met before we express needs for security. When these are met we recognize social needs, and so on up the pyramid to self-actualization. Health workers in deprived communities are familiar with families struggling with the fact that, to provide food for their families, they must give less priority to housing. For those with inadequate housing, they may have enough food but may place housing needs before preventive health needs. We might conclude that we view our needs differently in different circumstances, and that needs have an important subjective element. This is before we consider whether these needs may or may not be met by health care.

Just as the idea of need seems more complex than at first glance, so too is the idea of health. The World Health Organization defines health as: *'a state of complete, physical, mental and social well being and not merely the absence of disease or infirmity'* (WHO 1978) and: *'the extent to which an individual or group is able to satisfy needs, realize aspirations and change or cope with their environment. Health is a resource for everyday life, not the objective of living; it is a positive concept, emphasizing social and personal resources as well as physical capabilities'* (WHO 1981).

By these broad definitions, health needs include maximizing the capabilities of people to function within their own limits and cultures, and could include a poor standard of living, in that it interferes with mental and social well-being – aside from the known impact of inadequate housing, unsafe transport and diet, on health. Too often the term 'needs assessment' is assumed to relate only to health care needs assessment, when a range of environmental and social needs dwarf the potential impact of

formal health care. The ability to use new information systems to integrate the perceptions of social scientists with practice management, clinical decision making and resource allocation has been described by Fitzpatrick (1994) as a revolution. But he tempers this by pointing out that we should be cautious in incorporating health status measurement into local population surveys. After all, we do not know how we should translate population health status into actual services. How much health care does any given health problem require? Health profiling, a way of bringing together qualitative and quantitative information about a community (which may be relevant to the community's health), is more of an attempt to validate local health care provision than a health needs assessment in itself (see Ch. 11). Provocatively, Frankel (1991) describes this activity as a professionally reassuring displacement activity in a time of uncertainty. But he also stresses the invalidity of making resource allocation decisions from measures of need based on the use of deprivation indices – such measurements of social need are no quick fix for the assessment of health needs (see Ch. 8).

Patients do not present themselves for consultation with a diagnostic label which says they have diabetes or need an operation. Most present with symptoms associated with their changing experience of life: they report work stress, marital problems; they provide psychosomatic cues such as headaches or bowel disturbance. Insomnia and loss of self-esteem cover a myriad of problems, some of which have clear causes and some of which do not. Of UK general practice consultations, 46% are 'minor', of which a quarter are minor psychoemotional or unexplained symptoms; a third of all consultations involve significant social problems (Fry 1995). What is clear is that in order to address the broader aspects of people's health in primary health care, we must define needs outside the traditional biomedical model of diseases and diagnoses. Diagnostic labels in (for example) mental health are poor indicators of need for education, support or employment. This approach is consistent with emerging psychological research which has linked social support, dispositional hostility and work strain to health outcomes (Adler & Mathews 1994).

General practitioners (GPs) might argue that their traditional skills have included listening to patients to discern their needs. Does this not suggest that all we have to do is ask people in order to assess their needs? Or why not simply look at the use of health services? Unfortunately there are some problems with these approaches. Firstly, the population which uses the services of a general practitioner is not representative of the population as a whole. If people believe that health services can help with their problem they will use health services; if they do not, then they may deal with it in some other way. For example, if it is believed that there is no useful treatment for migraine, people will not consult their GPs about migraine. Looking at those who use health services can simply reinforce what people already believe about health services and what services are available. The fact that a service is provided will tend to lead to its use. Secondly, there is a distinction between the needs of individuals and the needs of the community. An individual (or, in this case, a couple) may need an expensive infertility treatment, but to what extent does the community need them to have a child? Here we are also entering into the distinction between needs, wants and demands. The migraine sufferer needs relief, he may want relief also, but as he does not know that this want or need can be met, he does not seek relief by using the health services. His need is unexpressed. Economists, more familiar with economic evaluation and concepts of demand than need, are scornful of 'needologists' as they fail to show how needs assessments would affect resource allocation. Williams (1992) argues that the very word 'need' encourages a black and white approach to decision making, which distracts from the basic task of prioritizing competing claims. Many GPs would probably be happy without either economic evaluations or needs assessments; managers are generally more enthusiastic to be informed by needs assessment, but public health specialists are often doubtful that the process can be carried out within managerial time and resource constraints.

It helps to remember why this process is being embarked upon at all. The key aim of needs assessment is to answer a question, 'what are we doing (for our population of potential patients) and what should we be doing?' In the end this is a question for anyone who works in the health service.

DEFINITIONS AND SCOPE

Need	The potential to benefit from care
Demand	Expressed need for services accessible and purchasable by or for the demander
Supply	Services that are actually provided

Need

Need is far from being a simple concept, and discussion of health needs is complicated by a variety of differing approaches to the subject. These derive from different professional understandings of the concept. The aim of this section is to spell out some of these and to show how they relate to each other.

One of the most widely used models of need derives from Bradshaw (1972). In it, a distinction is made between felt, expressed, normative and comparative needs (Box 1.1). A second way of looking at need is provided by Stevens & Gabbay (1991), who differentiate between need, demand and supply (Fig. 1.2).

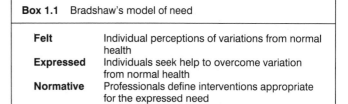

Box 1.1	Bradshaw's model of need
Felt	Individual perceptions of variations from normal health
Expressed	Individuals seek help to overcome variation from normal health
Normative	Professionals define interventions appropriate for the expressed need
Comparative	Comparison between needs using severity, size, range of interventions, etc., usually between similar locations

A third contribution to the discussion derives from an economic model of behaviour, which emphasizes that needs are relative and depend on individual circumstances. Unfortunately, some of the confusion around the subject arises from the fact that different authors use the same terminology to mean different things.

Need is best thought of as the potential to benefit from health care. A person who has a problem which could be alleviated by a medical intervention is in need. The

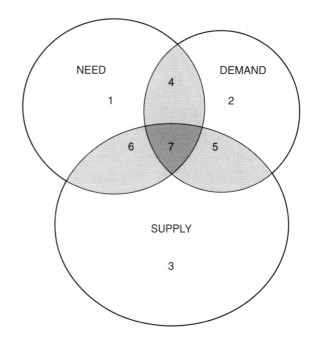

Figure 1.2 Another way of looking at need, differentiating it from demand and supply.

Examples of these in a district might be:-

1. A stroke unit
2. Circumcision
3. Routine antenatal checks
4. Early physiotherapy in acute back pain
5. Antibiotics for viral upper respiratory tract infection
6. Hearing aids for the elderly
7. Inhaled therapies for asthma

(Adapted, with permission, from Stevens (1991).)

intervention could be treatment, advice or simply diagnostic or prognostic information. In some cases this is fairly uncontroversial: both the patient and the clinician agree. If I have appendicitis, I believe I need surgery and so does my doctor. But if I go to my GP with a self-limiting condition, I probably think of myself as in need, but my GP may not agree. Similarly, my GP may decide that I need advice on my alcohol consumption, or a blood pressure measurement, but I may not agree. This illustrates two divergent concepts of need, *self-perceived need* (felt need) and *normative need*. The former I decide for myself; the latter is determined by a health professional, who decides according to professional norms (hence 'normative').

Each has different implications. Self-perceived need is dependent on my knowledge and understanding of what health care can do for me. This has the advantage that I know myself and I am able to judge just how much of a problem a symptom is to me and what priority it should receive in my circumstances. However, it has the disadvantage that I may not know much about illnesses and what might be of use in treating them. Normative need, on the other hand, is dependent on the opinion and knowledge of the doctor. It can be influenced by factors which affect these, such as training, specific areas of skill or interest, method of remuneration and so on. It is also, more fundamentally, influenced by professional beliefs about what is a legitimate health problem and what is not. Underlying this distinction is a more philosophical question: who is the best judge of my interests? The assumption of a normative view of need is that a professional is often the best judge of my interests; the assumption of a self-perceived view of need is that I myself am the best judge.

A further complication arises when a normative view of need reflects the needs of the community. This may be in conflict with my perception of my (felt) need. Compulsory psychiatric care is an obvious example of this, but there are more subtle instances: parents who decline to have their children immunized, thereby putting other children at risk of contracting infectious diseases, or people who do not wear a seat-belt in the car, and run the risk of costing the health service more if they crash. Indeed, the fact that we offer 'free' health care (at the point of use) but not free televisions or holidays is a reflection of the fact that as a community we feel a need to provide the former but not the latter. In each of these cases we can distinguish between what the individual patient wants and what the doctor or community wants for the patient. Spek (1972) devised a classification in which needs are judged by society, experts and individuals; and assessed by answering two question, 'Is the individual sick?' and 'Is the individual in need of public health care?'

Demand

Demand is a concept more usually associated with economics. In the context of health care, demand is taken to mean a need which has led to some action in search of health care. This is called *expressed need* by Bradshaw. For a need to be expressed, two conditions must be met. Firstly I must perceive that I have a need – in other words there must be a felt need – and, further, I must have the means to do something about it. If the service which I feel I need is inaccessible to me, too expensive for me or I do not know about it, then my need may not be expressed. Apparently I have no demand for such a service. Yet, if I acquire the means to do something about my felt need, I may start to express a need: now I apparently do have a demand. This may seem contradictory. A look at an economic model may help to clarify matters.

In economics, demand is a measure of desire for something. When we talk about demand, then, we are talking about strength of desire. The strength of desire is measured in terms of what we would be prepared to give up in order to get it. In health care we usually give up time and money (consultation fees in a private system, but also travel costs or prescription fees in the National Health Service (NHS)), to gain access to a service. This is called the *opportunity cost*. Different people will value a service (such as a consultation with a doctor) differently, but, overall, fewer will want the service if the opportunity cost is high, than if it is low. In other words, demand (or expressed need) is not a fixed quantity, but is dependent on the opportunity cost. If a service is free and easily accessible, more will express a need (there will be more demand) for it than if it is costly and inaccessible. Put another way, we cannot say that the demand for a health service is X, we can only say that *given the current pattern of provision* the demand is X.

Another factor which influences our demand for health care hinges on the phrase 'have the means to do something about it'. In a private system, those with more disposable income tend to use health care more. Those for whom health insurance pays more of the cost of treatment will also demand more as, in effect, it costs them less. In a 'free' health service such as the NHS, the means to do something may be largely knowledge of the service and how to access it.

Supply

Supply refers to the health care services which are available, what we actually provide. Inevitably, this is a reflection of more than simply need or even demand, because historical or political factors play an important role. An example of this is the way in which traditional professional boundaries determine the services which we are able to provide within the NHS. It might be useful from the point of view of the back-pain sufferer directly to see a manipulative therapist who could prescribe painkillers, issue a sickness certificate, take radiographs and refer to a specialist if necessary. This would be difficult in view of the traditional separation of professional responsibility for prescribing, manipulative therapy, sickness certification and referral. In this case, history and legal definitions of professions determine the nature of the service supplied.

COMMISSIONERS, PROVIDERS AND NEEDS ASSESSMENT

Since the NHS reforms, two distinct functions of the health service have been separated. On the one hand are commissioners or purchasers, who must decide what services they should commission for the population. This is done within the limits of a fixed budget for a fixed population. Contracts are written with providers of health care, which might be hospitals (either privately or publicly owned), clinicians (for example GPs) or other professionals. In theory, the commissioner is not obliged to contract with any particular provider, but to act in the best interest of the population. The emphasis on contracting may be unfortunate, as it is not clear that it is a good way of bringing about change in clinical practice. More attention is now being given to other aspects of commissioning such as influencing opinion leaders or local government, training and purchasing development programmes or evaluations. These are much more important in the UK primary care system.

Needs assessment is seen by commissioners (health authority or fundholding general practice) as a means of deciding how the service provision it purchases should change. In practice, because purchasing health care through contracts is unwieldy, the transaction costs are high and the costs of providing health care are not accurately known, the process of changing contracts is fraught with operational problems. Most services are contracted on historical patterns, changed only at the margins, with little information about needs. But service development is more likely to be guided by needs assessment in the future, to avoid the situation where professional providers of health care dominate service changes at the expense of consumers or the population as a whole. Needs assessment has traditionally been regarded as falling into three categories: corporate (see Chs 8 and 10), comparative (see Chs 7 and 8) and epidemiologically based (see Ch 6) (Box 1.2). It is not clear whether this classification is sufficient, and a broader functional approach is used in this book. Only the corporate methods have tended to be integrated into commissioning.

Box 1.2 Traditional classification of needs assessment

1. Epidemiological
- **Ideal** – involves developing and using an instrument to detect and measure individuals who will benefit from an intervention, measuring demand, and applying to specific populations

  Impractical except as a research and development tool

- **Pragmatic** – involves triangulation of:
  - estimation of incidence and prevalence
  - summary of services available
  - identification of effective interventions

2. Comparative
- How does provision in district A compare with another population?
- Involves standardization and regression if being quantified

  Inaccurate, but it may be the only feasible technique. If nothing else is known about the best service to provide, there is an indication of need for further investigation, if local services differ markedly from the norm

3. Corporate
- Loose term describing synthesis of views of interested parties, to give credibility and accountability to decisions

  In common usage in health authorities who greatly value GPs' own views, but rarely says anything about need. GP purchasers would do well to take account of other contributors, including patients and the health authority

---

THE AGENCY RELATIONSHIP

If the relationship between purchaser and provider is determined by contracts, what is the relationship between patients and GPs? One way of looking at this is the agency relationship. As health is an area where we prefer not to learn by trial and error, and health services are complex to the outsider, we generally rely on the advice of our GP. The GP decides what is wrong and advises on a course of action (whether watchful waiting, treatment or referral). The GP is acting as an agent on the patient's behalf. In an idealized form, the GP always acts in the patient's interests and only in those interests. If the patient is not satisfied, he can look for another GP.

In terms of our model of need, demand and supply, the GP is a means of translating the patient's *demand* into a professional view of what the patient could benefit from: *normative need*. There are, however, certain tensions in the agency relationship.

Firstly, there may be incentives for the GP to influence the patient's demand in a way which is not in his interest – there are financial incentives to undertreat or overtreat. This has been demonstrated in the USA, where referrals to hospital are considerably less numerous under insurance schemes where the health maintenance organization (which employs the referring doctors) bears the cost from its own budget, compared with schemes where the insurer bears the cost independently of the referring doctor (Newhouse 1993). In the former case, the doctor has an incentive to consider the cost of inpatient treatment, but none in the latter.

Secondly, the GP may take a broader view of health than simply dealing with the patient in front of him. He may recognize, for example, that if all smokers in a practice population stop, there would be considerably less health disease, and may advise accordingly. However, for any one patient, there is no guarantee that this advice will be of benefit. Some will not suffer ill effects from their smoking; others may be unlucky and become ill whether they stop or not. Only some will have ill health prevented by giving up. Individuals may respond to this advice differently, some will stop smoking, while others will reason that it is not worth the effort. The doctor and the patient's view of what is needed may diverge. They might alternatively limit their prescribing or referral in order to encourage self-care and reduce the potential for 'somatic fixation' or to encourage a more appropriate use of resources. In either case, there is potential for conflict between the 'public good' and what the patient perceives as his immediate best interests.

COMMISSIONING

In this framework of commissioners and providers, primary care is in an interesting position. In the NHS, it is GPs who are contracted to provide the bulk of primary care (either themselves of through their attached staff). In a primary care-led NHS, one of the principal aims is to bring the level of decision making closer to patients. Another is to strengthen relationships between primary care and commissioning. For GPs this will mean involvement in strategic purchasing decisions in their area. It is important to realize that other primary care providers (for example, social workers, community-based nurses, and midwives) also have a role to play in this respect. GPs are clearly providers of health care as they directly care for patients. GPs who hold budgets are also purchasers, since they are responsible for commissioning some secondary care and other services for their patients. However, *all* GPs have two roles in the health service which lend themselves to purchasing. GPs are, for most patients, the first point of contact with the health services; in addition, they are responsible for access to a great many of the other services (the 'gatekeeper' function). Since clinical decisions taken by the GP determine what services each patient will use, it makes sense for GPs to have a say in deciding what services patients need.

Traditionally, GPs have tended to follow the practice and leadership of specialists in deciding referral patterns, clinical management and prescribing. The post-reform NHS has challenged this, and primary care doctors have the opportunity to shape decision making

around a primary care view of the service. This means that the pattern of secondary care and priorities in spending will be guided by what general practice and their community colleagues feel makes sense in the context of the wider health problems of the community. This is very different from the traditional approach of hospital consultants, who tend to define priorities by starting from the diseases they see and the high-technology tools they enjoy.

Health authorities up to now have used Maxwell's principles (Box 1.3). Primary care may view these differently, and suggested principles have been put forward by Harris (1996) for commissioning of and by primary care. These are shown in Box 1.4

Box 1.3 Maxwell's dimensions of quality

Effectiveness
Efficiency
Equity
Accessibility
Social acceptability
Relevance to need

Box 1.4 Harris's principles for commissioning

For commissioning of primary care:
　　Appropriateness (which site, (which) professional, standard of
　　　care)
　　Value for money
　　Patient empowering (health education, reducing demand for
　　　and utilization of services)
　　Social acceptability
　　Accessibility
　　Maximization of evidence-based practice
For commissioning of secondary care by primary care:
　　Maximization of effectiveness and monitoring of outcomes
　　Equity (geographic, client, type of purchaser)
　　Social acceptability
　　Efficiency
　　Responsiveness to primary care
　　Reflecting epidemiologically based need

WHOSE VALUES AND PRIORITIES?

Essentially, theories of distributive justice guide our decisions, often implicitly (we instinctively think it is fair). But it is important for those involved in resource allocation decisions to be more explicit about their underlying values. Some examples are given in Table 1.1.

The crucial position of equity in the jigsaw of resource allocation and the different approaches to understanding it cannot be divorced from the process of needs assessment. Needs assessment is itself a means of addressing an equity goal. Indeed, one economist holds that need is simply an incomplete criterion for using equity to choose between different patterns of health

Table 1.1 Theories of distributive justice (Periera 1993)

Type	Comments
Needs based	Maintain normal functioning Equality of opportunity for normal functioning
Contractarian	From behind a veil of ignorance, individuals decide on the basis of their needs based on the assumption that they might find themselves in the place of the worst off. In practice it means giving the highest priority to those in worst health
Egalitarian	Equality, regardless of needs
Entitlement	Equity is judged on the basis of 'just deserts'. Most health or illness is seen as equitable because it results from individuals' own decisions. For the state to interfere with this is inequitable. Only ill health resulting from genetic accident or inflicted by another person should be addressed by the state
Utilitarian	Maximizes the benefit to the whole community, irrespective of who benefits, rich or poor, healthy or ill, deserving or undeserving

service provision (Culyer 1995). His (abridged) criteria for needs assessment suggest that they are never all present, which may cast doubt on the value of the whole process (Box 1.5). Let us look at some of these. For needs (defined as a capacity to benefit from health care) to be a useful concept, there must be sufficient epidemiological information to identify the beneficiaries. Clearly the application of knowledge about needs may increase inequity for some groups. For example, health education tends to further advantage the advantaged, who already enjoy better health. Horizontal equity aims to treat those with the same need equally, vertical equity is the aim of allocating more to those with greatest need. These aims may conflict. We can aim for equity in resource allocation (in the UK, at present Scotland and London are at relative advantage in these terms), but this may not translate into equity in provision. Service use has been adopted as an equity goal, but we do not know how this reflects patient need: how much is inappropriate use or how much potential utilization is deterred by the pattern of provision. Equality of access may be a better equity goal, but its implementation may involve diverting resources from those receiving care to those who at present do not. Losers in this process may be better able to articulate their losses than potential gainers are able to

Box 1.5 Culyer's criteria for needs assessment

1. The values underlying needs assessment should be explicit
2. It is derived from the objective of the health system
3. It can be applied in practice to all members of the community (horizontal distribution) and all degrees of ill health (vertical distribution)
4. It must specify which service and which users are its target
5. It has a straightforward link to resources
6. It should not lead to inequitable results when applied to resource distribution

make a case for their gains. It is easy to produce plans or strategies with many principles, and conflicting equity goals. These are only useful if there is a way of linking the principles and values, through needs assessment to the process of resource allocation (see Ch. 8).

If general practice fails to grasp the nettle, others will continue to make priorities based on their own values. These combine the results of historic service provision with the influence of the best placed pressure groups. There are several lessons from this. Needs assessment may shape policy. The process has to address the issue of resource allocation if it is to be anything other than an academic exercise. Finally, there must be guiding principles and values. This raises the question of whose values. And how those values might be reflected.

Various initiatives have been taken to develop local voices in prioritizing local services (Winkler 1996). Lessons from these include the technical problems of obtaining a representative sample and the wording of questions; gaps in knowledge of expected benefits of services; problems when applying the findings; the reluctance of some of the public to take responsibility for the decisions. In Oregon, a variety of utilitarian and needs-based approaches were used to prioritize services to be paid for under the state Medicaid programme. The aim was that, by reducing the range of treatments offered, a wider number of people could be offered Medicaid cover. But some of the decisions reached by the process were overruled by health policy makers (often on the grounds of public health interest), and the process was bedevilled by the accusation that most of the public meetings were packed with health care professionals. In the NHS, even rationing of services of dubious effectiveness (many grommet insertions) or of low relevance to the population (tattoo removal or infertility treatments) tend to lead to an outcry.

The real lesson is that it is probably mistaken to ask others to advise on difficult decisions for which one is responsible. It is better to gain local public acceptance about the principles upon which decisions should be based and on the criteria which should be followed in their implementation. If this were combined with robust techniques for monitoring health services, and measuring preferences and outcomes, a public decision-making process could be informed by valid information. A better form of public accountability is needed than what we have at present, if we are to find a more acceptable way of using the public resources of the NHS effectively and justly.

Gaining public acceptance is time-consuming and difficult. In high-publicity cases in the UK, where the health authority attempts to restrict purchase of some procedures, it is often the public health doctor who is paraded in support of management, giving a professional or medical view about the proposed policy or action. This has brought public health doctors into a position between clinicians, the public and management. It is useful, then, to consider these roles, as understanding them is crucial to judging the value of needs assessment.

PUBLIC HEALTH MEDICINE AND GENERAL PRACTICE

Public health medicine is a discipline, built on a traditional consultant and junior doctor hierarchy, with its own faculty, and is sometimes confusingly referred to as 'public health', which term is used by a range of non-medical professions, managers and researchers often working closely with public health physicians to describe their field of work. The public health function in the NHS is medically led by the Chief Medical Officer, and the Department of Health views public health expertise as central to making these priority resource allocation decisions. Its role was defined in the Acheson Report (DH 1988) as 'the science and art of preventing disease, prolonging life and promoting health, through organised efforts of society'. The successor Abrams Report (DH 1993) stresses that 'the prime responsibility of the NHS is to maintain and improve the health of the population; this public health function underpinning all NHS purchaser and provider activity; all constituent parts of the NHS have a responsibility to demonstrate that their activities contribute to this aim' and that district directors of public health should 'provide the focus for a comprehensive public health strategy'.

General practice has been defined by the Royal College of General Practitioners (RCGP) as far back as 1972 (RCGP 1972) as 'personal, primary and continuing medical care to individuals and families ... [the doctor] will intervene educationally, preventively and therapeutically to promote his patient's health'. With the growth in preventive activities such as elderly screening and child immunization and surveillance in general practice, and the GMS contractual commitment to chronic disease management, there has been an increasing health promotional role in general practice. The requirement for the first time that fundholders should address in their practice plan their contribution to national targets (NHS Executive 1995) also shows the converging of the roles of public health and primary health care.

Much of the current confusion about professional roles is due to the historical development of each discipline in the NHS. Tudor-Hart (1984) has observed that 'community medicine will take time to recover from a century of banishment to the periphery of medical practice, but clinicians will also take time to recover from their ignorance of the tasks of organisation, management, local planning, and research based clinical strategy'. Does the current focus on commissioning effective clinical interventions based on needs assessment represent the recovery of both disciplines? Or is this a managerial pipe dream, far removed from the realities of practice? There is evidence of great interest in collaboration between the two disciplines in infectious disease control, audit, evaluation, pharmacoeconomics and contract specification, but less evidence of widespread joint working. Bhopal (1995) has pointed out that whilst deficits in skills and knowledge can be overcome by hard work, the differing perspectives and attitudes of public health doctors (population, environment, prevention, and society) and general practitioners (individual patients, the consultation, medical interventions and care of the sick) are incompatible. The different approaches to achieving the same goal have been described by Bhopal (Table 1.2).

This analysis highlights the different approaches of the disciplines, which need to be understood, to conduct needs assessment (see Ch. 2). However, it disguises the role conflicts in each, which create great tension, particularly in relationship to management, and the changing structure of the NHS. Harris (1995) has described these (Table 1.3). For example, in addressing the need to develop a service, the public health doctor may be pulled between his corporate responsibility to the cash-limited health authority, who may not view it as a priority, and his professional independent role to be an advocate for the needs of the population. At the same time, the GP has a tension between responsibility to the needs of his practice, and its population, and the individual patients who present to him. This leads to consideration of reducing conflicts of interests, which may be essential if needs assessment is to lead to service development. One way is to separate out the roles between different individuals in the same organization (e.g. between practice manager and partner) or by reversing current trends of convergence, by separating out conflicting roles in different organizations (between the GP and public health of doctor). A more innovative way has been explored by the King's Fund (King's Fund

Table 1.2 Different approaches to public health

Public health approach	Agenda	Primary care approach
Evaluation of structure process and outcome of services	*Effectiveness and efficiency of services*	Clinical Audit and Practice organization
Based primarily on epidemiological and demographic data, and economic concepts		Based partly on subjective views of staff and patients
Emphasis on needs of those who make no demand	*Assessment of health needs*	Based mainly on demands of patients and contractual obligations

Reproduced, with permission, from Bhopal (1995).

Table 1.3 Potential conflicts in roles

Executive Public Health Medicine role	Partner in General Practitioner role
accountability to the Health Authority v. the local community	accountability to the practice population v. the individual patient
public corporate responsibility v. professional independence	practice responsibility (e.g. to service development) v. individual patient care
present pragmatist v. future strategist	proactive and preventative care v. reactive patient care
self censorship v. consumer advocacy	relying on self assessment of priorities (e.g. in care rationing) v. individual patient advocacy
role in health authority management structure v. consultant status	role in relation to practice manager v. GP principal status
medical v. non medical public health practitioners	GP role as employer v. autonomy PHCT, e.g. developing nurse practitioners/therapy contractors
use of executive power v. influence on clinician opinion leaders	use of political power v. peer influence and education
advice to health authority purchaser v. advice to GP fundholder purchaser	role as GP fundholder purchaser v. role as GP provider
responsibilty for population normative need v. expressed need and demand	responsibility to use normative clinical standards (e.g. guidelines) v. response to patient demand
utilitarianism v. equity of opportunity in resource allocation	services to provide the greatest good overall v. accessibility of care (esp. minority groups)

Table 1.4 Possible future GP roles

Role	Responsibilities
Clinical servant	Clinical care, professional education and clinical research
Health councillor	Patient advocate and personal decision consultant, lobbyist, networker
Chief executive officer	Corporate expression general practice, contracts and service agreements
Care shaper	Change agent across boundaries, service development manager

Adapted, with permission, from King's Fund (1995).

1995), that is, to create new roles within general practice (Table 1.4).

The care shaper could be a dually trained public health doctor and GP or a specialist change agent with a background of primary care practice and public health attitudes. He could develop the technical skills to monitor and assess need in practice or locality populations, and perhaps address the broader needs of people outside the health sector (see Ch. 10). Indeed, the fact that there are 30 times more GPs than public health doctors shows the importance of GPs incorporating the public health perspectives and skills within their teams, rather than relying on external help. Such ideas serve to stress the importance of being explicit about and understanding each other's roles, and in the long-term generating new joint working through training initiatives, the annual public health report and commissioning, if needs assessment is to be fruitful.

The RCGP report 'The nature of general medical practice' (RCGP 1996) recognizes these tensions and opportunities, and highlights another – that between the art and science of medical practice. It urges sole professional control of its activity, without identifying how that is possible with greater public accountability. The difficulty in primary care for GPs in embracing needs

assessment, like the difficulty of public health doctors in giving priority to demand management, partly reflects the organizational constraints of each other's workplace. Forward-looking general practices are giving priority to the art of designing and managing a type of primary care organization of the future. It should remain professionally led, and stay sufficiently small and approachable, and yet use effectively local community networks, and work within a system of public servant accountability. This is complex and needs skilled management. Forward-thinking public health physicians have raised their vision from the priority of supporting commissioning in health authorities to the opportunities of change management, health care evaluation, health promotion, population advocacy, professional education and service development outside. New organizational working arrangements may emerge in provider units, general practice consortia, academic units, consultancies, local government, voluntary sectors, the media, and consumer organizations. Above all, there needs to be a sharing of skills, between general practice and public health specialists. We all need to grow our organizations to fit our purposes, and not to tailor our work to fit our organizations.

MANAGEMENT AND MEDICINE

How are we to design and run our organizations to promote health? Here we need skills of managers, too often vilified for executing exceptionally challenging tasks. An American doctor commented on the conflict in the NHS between the medical profession and management, soon after the introduction of the NHS reforms thus (Sabin 1992).

'Embracing traditional collective responsibilities and the new consumerism will create too much tension for comfort. . . A visitor can only hope that you in Britain will be more successful than we in the United States have been at distinguishing principles that should be fought for, from habits and vested interests that may be painful to relinquish, but do not reflect the ethical core of medicine.'

Needs assessment may be cynically seen at best as an irrelevance, at worst as a threatening management tool, giving a scientific basis to irresponsible consumerism.

The studies of Delbecq and Gill (1985) show the different behaviours of physicians and managers under threat; physicians do not respond to a hierarchical structure, and become more autonomous, whilst managers of large organizations become more cohesive, seeking maximum influence on others. This creates a barrier to achieving any change. Managers are often criticized by the clinical professions for short-termism and failing to close the gap between intent and implementation (Pettigrew 1986). Best has identified some common organizational pathologies that underlie this (Best 1986). First is the tendency for managerial accountability to be task based, promoting short-term visible results at long-term expense. The second is the overemphasis on statements of strategic intent, such as the detailed ambitious health strategies of health authorities, with insufficient attention to the organization's capacity to deliver. Thirdly is an excessive focus on organizational process, losing vision and sensitivity to external factors.

All three of these organizational pathologies may be eased by needs assessment. Needs assessment provides a mechanism for managers to focus on longer-term strategic issues, often ones on which doctors have been urging action. Through a process of needs assessment doctors can bring their unique insights without being hastily prejudged as voicing vested interests. Secondly needs assessment focuses on the detail and complexity of providing health care and promoting health. It inevitably produces much information, which tempers over ambitious strategic intentions and focuses the managerial eye on the constraints and processes of achieving change to meet that need. The third pathology is remedied by the very nature of needs assessment, reaching out to the community and the determinants of health, which refocuses the organization on its purpose, when it is preoccupied with its own incremental changes.

Good managerial skills have never been more needed, both in the large NHS organizations and in small practices and departments. Knowing more about needs should be a resource for general practitioners, managers and public health specialists alike. Needs assessment should be the ground on which the professions, management and consumers all meet. In any democratic society there will be tensions between these groups. Needs driven policy creates opportunities for rational and open consideration of options and practices. To have fruitful discussions we must understand each other's language and not just be the mouthpiece of our tribal language. Needs, demand, strategy, public health – all have different meanings to different people. It is hoped that those engaged in the worthy pursuit of promoting the health of our population will find common languages. Eloise, over time, had made her meaning crystal clear when she stated 'I need a hug'. Perhaps the most important lesson for all on working with others in the health service is to ask what others mean, before we form a view. The language of needs assessment is fraught with misunderstandings. Incidentally, I wonder what the NHS workplace would be like if we were all a little more honest to each other in stating our individual needs.

REFERENCES

Adler N, Mathews K 1994 Health psychology: why do some people get sick and some stay well? Annual Review of Psychology 45: 229–259

Best G 1986 Strategic managing, organizational learning and development strategy Ch 12: Managers as strategists, Persten G. King's Fund, London

Bhopal R S 1995 Public health medicine and primary health care: convergent. Divergent or parallel paths? Epidemiology and Community Health 49: 116–133

Bradshaw J 1972 A taxonomy of social need problems and progress in medical care. Seventh series: Nuffield Provincial Hospitals Trust, Oxford University Press, Oxford

Bradshaw J 1994 The conceptualisation and measurement of need. A social policy perspective. Ch 3: Researching people's health. Popay & Williams, Routledge

Cole G A 1993 Management: theory and practice. Major theories of human motivation 4th Edition. DP Publications, London

Culyer A J 1995 Need: the idea won't do – but we still need it. Editorial. Soc Sci Med Vol 40; 6: 727–730

Delbecq A L, Gill S L 1985 Justice as a prelude to teamwork in medical centres. Healthcare Management Review. US

Department of Health 1988 Public health in England. The Acheson Report. Cmd paper 289

Department of Health November 1993 Public health: responsibilities of the NHS and the roles of others. Advice of the committee set up to undertake a review of HC (88) 64 (The Abrams Report) Accompanying HSG (93) 56 NHSE

Fitzpatrick R 1994 Health needs assessment Ch 10: Chronic illness and the social sciences Researching people's health. Popay & Williams Routledge

Frankel S 1991 The epidemiology of indications. Epidemiology and Community Health; 45: 257–259

Fry 1995 Reviving primary care. A US-UK comparison, Fry, Light, Rodnick, Orton, Radcliffe Medical Press

Hadoran D C 1991 The role of public values in setting health care priorities. Soc Sci Med Vol 32; 7: 773–781

Harris A 1995 Freshfields. The relationship between public health medicine and general medical practice. Primary care Management 5 No. 7

Harris A 1996 Making sense of a primary care NHS. Ch 2: Primary care policy. Radcliffe Medical Press

Hauser M The economics of medical care. Allen & Unwin, London

Huygen F J A, Mokkink H G A, Smiths A J A et al 1992 Relationship between working styles of general practitioners and the health status of their patients. British Journal of General Practice 42: 144–149

King's Fund 1995 Exploring new roles in general practice: a day in the life of a GP 2010. King's Fund Centre Workshops

Newhouse 1993 Free for all? Lessons from the Rand experiment. Harvard University Press

NHS Executive November 1995 EL (95) 54. An accountability framework for GP fundholding. Leeds

Periera J 1993 What does equity in health care mean? J. Social Policy; 22; 19–48

Pettigrew AM 1986 Managing strategic change Ch 9: Managers as strategists. Persten G. King's Fund, London

RCGP 1972 The future general practitioner, learning and teaching. Royal College of General Practitioners/BMJ, London

RCGP 1996 The nature of general medical practice. Report from general practice 27. Royal College of General Practitioners. London

Sabin JE 1992 Mind the gap. Reflections of an American health maintenance organizations doctor on the new NHS BMJ 305: 514–516

Spek JE 1972 The economic analysis of health and medical care in a Swedish health district Hauser M. The economics of medical care, Allen & Unwin, London

Stevens A, Gabbay J 1991 Needs assessment needs assessment. Health Trends 23: 20–23

Tudor-Hart J 1984 Community general practitioners. BMJ 288: 1670–1673

WHO 1978 Primary health care. Report of the International Conference on Primary Health Care, Alma-Ata, Geneva

WHO 1981 Halfdon-Mahler The meaning of health for all by the year 2000. World Health Forum 3 (1): 5–22

Williams 1992 Priorities not needs. Corden A, Robertson G, Tolley K. Meeting needs, Avebury Gower, Aldershot

Winkler F 1996 Involving patients: Ch 12. Meads G. A primary care-led NHS: putting it into practice, Churchill Livingstone, Edinburgh

2

How to get started

*Judith Hooper   Nigel Edwards
Sarah Ann Ujah*

The last chapter sought to illuminate what we mean by 'need'. This chapter seeks to throw light on what is meant by 'assessment'. It describes, from experience of working with general practice, the key steps in getting started, potential pitfalls and some tips on avoiding them or possible solutions. Probably the most crucial point to remember is that *health needs assessment (HNA) is about change, so stick to specifics and what is possible*; otherwise HNA can be demoralizing in its diversity and complexity.

WHAT IS HEALTH NEEDS ASSESSMENT AND WHY BOTHER?

The previous chapter has shown how health encompasses a diversity of influences: cultural, social, education, housing, transport and environmental. These all shape needs, which imply an ability to benefit. So assessment requires a clear definition of both the issue or problem and what can be done to benefit. This is done by identifying what the problem is, the factors affecting its distribution and impact on people, who has the problem and what can be done to alleviate it, i.e. modify these factors. This is then compared with an analysis of present service provision, to create a plan for change that is agreeable to the key participants. It is like going round the audit cycle.

So, HNA systematically reviews the potential for alleviation of any health or health related issue against current service provision resulting in a shared rationale, priority setting and a plan for change.

HNA is a major cultural shift in service planning. The shift is from planning based on historical activity to systematically reviewing both the content and delivery of services, resulting in a more effective service, closely reflecting needs. HNA is about change from reactive service-driven care to proactive and needs-led care. The flowchart in Figure 2.1 shows the relationship between HNA and delivery of health care in a needs-led National Health Service (NHS). Note the need to balance

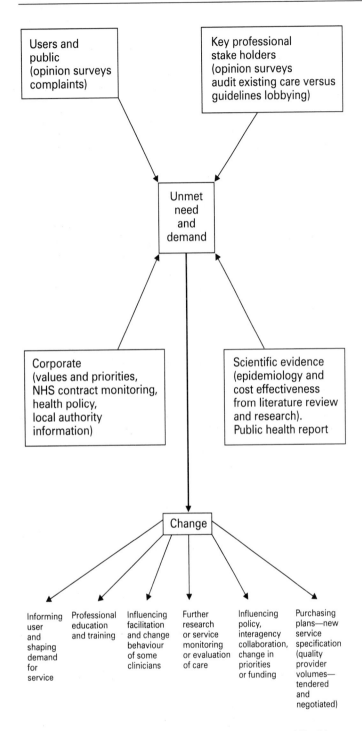

Figure 2.1 Framework for a needs-led NHS (Hooper and Harris).

Public opinion is useful and necessary for access and responsiveness of services (quality) but is likely to be distorted or limited in its ability to contribute to a debate about priorities, equity, effectiveness or efficiency. Where contracts are agreed without, or with, partial information from needs assessment, there is a high risk of providing inappropriate care.

The role of the primary health care team (PHCT) is to identify, prioritize and alleviate a wide diversity of needs, filtering patients to receive support or (secondary) services. Three basic public health principles are important for PHCTs in becoming needs led:

1. Assessments of health needs must be population based. Limitations and biases will be introduced if only current users are studied. Assessment of health of a practice population needs to cover distribution of diseases and problems, their impact or severity and identification of factors that modify these problems.

2. Health is much wider than health care. Promotion of health involves education, life style and information. Assessment of health should consider social risk factors and determinants, rehabilitation needs, disease screening and not just measurement of presented disease and treatments, i.e. all three levels of prevention.

3. It is important to recognize the legitimacy of the community and its identification of need (e.g. in terms of housing, transport and leisure). Concern for equity and social justice, knowing the perspectives and priorities of their community, are crucial in choosing and conducting appropriate needs assessments.

All of this will sound stratospheric to many PHCTs just about coping with their present workload. But the shift to a primary care-led NHS creates responsibilities and opportunities for PHCTs. In getting started it is much better to focus on what is within the control of the PHCT rather than cope with complex problems requiring multi-agency collaboration. Having completed the first HNA, then the team can move on to wider agendas identified from their practice diagnosis, the initial key step.

KEY STEPS

If the PHCT is unused to these steps then the team needs to gain knowledge and experience of them. A useful way is to pick a simple, well-defined health problem, for example asthma or a screening programme, and work through all the key steps for this problem, excluding the practice diagnosis and priority setting (Box 2.1). Alternatively, a key age group can be chosen (see Ch. 3). This will certainly help team building and reveal other skills or management systems in the PHCT that need improving, such as computer use and audit.

The key steps to successful health needs assessment are as follows:

professional perspectives, corporate and management views, scientific evidence and user's perceptions. Public opinion tends to support high technology and life-saving interventions at the cost of mental health and community services or particular minority groups or those with unfashionable conditions or who have some stigma. Information is often from serendipity and anecdote, especially from the media.

Box 2.1   Practical point

PHCTs probably already have issues that they wish to tackle. If PHCTs find the structure of HNA in its key steps new to them as a way of working, then they are better to choose a specific, well-defined issue they have control over, and leave both the practice diagnosis (step 2) and priority setting (step 3) until they have completed that HNA.

Box 2.2   Example

One PHCT took a different approach to team development (Adelaide Medical Centre Primary Health Care Team 1991). They drew up a manifesto which set aims, objectives and targets for all members of the team. This 'product definition' of the PHCT took over 2 years, and included the structure and process of the work of the team in its clinical and organizational aspects, emphasizing their independence. By developing the manifesto, real team work grew and their business plan was created, as well as being a means of constant review and amendment.

1. Ensure the PHCT functions as a *team*, can cope with change and can be flexible enough to change.

2. Given the diverse range of needs presenting to the PHCT, some system of information review about the practice population is needed, to identify the main problems. This is profiling the health of the practice population or *practice diagnosis*.

3. Given this range of issues, where does the PHCT start? The answer is to put the identified issues in an order of *priority*, agreeing criteria for this and applying them to each issue. This presents an explicit rationale for priority problems to be shared.

4. Define the *epidemiology* – the size, severity and population affected by the issue and factors influencing its distribution and impact.

5. Agree what should be *done* about the issue. Local knowledge and experience, experts and literature review should allow agreement as to what is effective and appropriate and what is not.

6. *Planning*:
   – Define a clear aim and objectives
   – Identify available skills, knowledge and resources and any gaps, and how to bridge them
   – Review what is being done now and how it is delivered
   – Identify changes needed between the present and what should be done (from step 5)
   – Agree an implementation plan of what will be done, how, by whom, when and where.

7. Choose appropriate *methods* of assessment, and manage information accordingly, i.e. plan data needs.

8. Work in partnership with *other agencies*.

9. Maintain *sustainability*, i.e. keep the process going.

STEP 1. IS THE PHCT FUNCTIONING AS A TEAM?

Primary health care needs a multidisciplinary team to achieve its role. If HNA is to be achieved in all its steps from practice diagnosis through to implementation plans for specific issues, then the pooling of knowledge, skills and experience of the team is essential (Box 2.2).

So *how well does the PHCT function?* Usually some part of the PHCT functions better than others. If this is a unidisciplinary part, e.g. nursing, general practitioners or administration staff, then it will be difficult to engage the whole PHCT. If this is a multidisciplinary part, then there is a much higher chance that the whole PHCT can be engaged because each professional group has a member involved with others as a team and can act as a bridge.

Are the definition and requirements of a team understood by each member?

What is a team?

A team is a group of people with *common objectives* who need to work together to achieve them. A team should

1. Support and help members
2. Coordinate activities
3. Generate commitment
4. Provide a sense of belonging, fulfilling a basic human need
5. Identify educational needs and learning opportunities
6. Enhance communication and understanding
7. Provide a satisfying, stimulating and enjoyable working environment
8. Achieve far more than the sum of its individual members.

A poorly functioning team will have at least some of the following characteristics:

1. Priorities are set by the most powerful, including the most vocal
2. The range of interventions and activities will be limited, undermining the definition of primary health care
3. Agreement on an appropriate skill mix will be limited and essential skills may be missing
4. Agreement on what should be done and who does what will be dictatorial, thus excluding ownership and increasing potential inefficiency
5. Lack of contribution will increase frustration and boredom
6. Duplication will occur as communication is poor
7. Boundaries will act as blocks, not as clarification

8. Mistakes will be used negatively as criticism, instead of being used as an opportunity for improvement.

Assessing individual perceptions of team functioning

A questionnaire that identifies the strengths and weaknesses of teams (Woodcock 1989) is provided in Appendix 1. A couple of hours is set aside for all the PHCT to work together, perhaps during a time out, with a skilled facilitator. Each PHCT member completes this questionnaire and the scoring. All responses are pooled onto a flipchart to 'eyeball' the range of answers. The ensuing discussion should give considerable insight and opportunities to improve team functioning, especially the contributions from members with outlying answers.

The PHCT could then try completing an HNA of an important problem to give a focus for enhancing team working, and then go to the practice diagnosis. This allows members who are team players to work up a concrete and real problem, over which the PHCT has some control, in order to motivate others.

Resources required

If the team needs some help in improving its functioning, some protected time led by an experienced facilitator in team building would be well worthwhile. Some management training for practice managers (and clinicians) can also be very useful. Health Authority primary care development staff should know sources of help and may be able to offer other resources such as funding or potential donors.

STEP 2. PRACTICE DIAGNOSIS

The PHCT need to pool available information about their population – health profiling or practice diagnosis (Table 2.1). From this, up to 10 issues are identified which are the most important for the PHCT population. The main reasons for going through this apparently lengthy process are:

1. To identify major health problems

Table 2.1 Sources of data for practice diagnosis

Potential routine practice data (see Ch. 4)

Age/sex	E.g. 0–4, 5–14, 15–24, 25–34, 35–44, 45–54, 55–64, 65–74, 75+ year age groups
Births	Total number, type of antenatal care, complications and type of delivery, birth weight under 2.5 kg
Children	Number on the Child Protection At Risk Register Immunization rates for children
Contraception	Number of women using the various methods Number of pregnancies in those aged under 16 years Number of terminations of pregnancies
Deaths	By cause, sex and age (e.g. under 65, 65–74, 75+ years old) Place of death: home, hospital, residential care (including hospice), other
Repeat prescribing	Prevalence of some diseases Costs of drugs
Health service use	PHCT of consultations (all types) Referrals to other agencies Hospital outpatient/inpatient episodes

Routine data from Public Health Information Departments of the Health Authority (see Ch. 12)

Census	Number of people living alone, single parents, ethnicity, car ownership, housing type, limiting long-term illness, unemployment: by ED, ward, practice
Communicable disease	Number of notifications by disease and age (e.g. 0–4, 5–14, 15–64, 65+ years old)
Child health surveillance	
Screening	Cervical and breast cancers: percentage ceased, uptake by age group Antenatal care

Specific information from practice (see Ch. 4 and Ch. 11)

Illness/prevalence	Acute and chronic Levels of functioning/complications
Health behaviours	Smokers Alcohol misusers Drug misusers
Registers	Screening programmes Chronic disease management – diabetes, asthma, ischaemic heart disease, etc.
Guidelines	Prescribing Programmes of care for chronic disease management
Audit results	
Other characteristics of area	Quality of housing, transport systems, shopping facilities, access to recreation areas, number of residential or nursing homes, etc.
Vulnerable people	Number of homeless, in B & B accommodation or hostels, travellers

---

Box 2.3 Key elements of a team (Woodcock 1989)

- Balanced roles
- Clear objectives and agreed targets for action
- Openness and ability to cope with confrontation
- Support and trust
- Cooperation and ability to cope with conflict
- Sound procedures
- Appropriate leadership
- Regular review
- Individual development
- Sound intergroup relations
- Good communications.

---

2. To ensure you do not inadvertently choose an issue of lower priority because it is currently the most obvious one
3. To avoid duplication of effort
4. To avoid ignoring an issue because the PHCT feels it is not a problem or not understood.

Sounding out to others, such as users, the local public health department, the Community Health Council (CHC), relevant voluntary groups, a local trust or another practice can be very helpful in checking perceptions. External agencies will have major priorities too, such as:

- *National*. Health of the Nation, the annual Priorities and Planning Guidance of the Department of Health.
- *Local*. Health authority purchasing intentions, based on local priorities for agreement with other providers. This will include areas of particular pressure, e.g. if there are long waiting times for orthopaedic out-patient assessments, then how many actually do not need surgery but effective interventions provided by alternative services such as physiotherapists or osteopaths? Initial measurement may identify this as a priority area for HNA.

Such consultation will save a lot of resources. It is often useful to profile the issues briefly at first then recheck the profile, including different information, after completing each health needs assessment.

A specific problem is identifying issues about which the PHCT has little control but might influence other agencies such as local authorities. A problem can often arise from not understanding the culture and centres of power within other agencies rendering any influence impotent, e.g. housing issues. Until the PHCT has experience of HNA, it may be better to stick to issues directly controlled to a considerable extent by the PHCT.

STEP 3. AGREE CRITERIA FOR SETTING ORDER OF PRIORITY FOR THESE ISSUES

HNA must remain manageable. The temptation to be sidetracked by the diversity of issues should be resisted as this diminishes the likelihood of real resultant benefit. To identify the main paths requires a list of preferred destinations, i.e. a list of issues in order of priority. To stick to the main paths requires a clear view of where you want to be, i.e. your objectives. How you get there, e.g. by auditing practice against guidelines, should be laid out in explicit implementation plans.

Criteria need to be agreed by the PHCT and applied consistently to all issues, including any weighting (Box 2.4).

Finally, is the choice of issue consistent with the priorities and objectives of the practice as a whole (Box 2.5)? If it is, then is there widespread ownership for change in the PHCT?

Feasibility

This includes both motivation and resources such as skills or time. The health problem may have a clearly defined population group who are contactable, based on geography, disease, socioeconomic, service use or other. Should the assessment review all that group or would a sample be sufficient and an efficient use of limited resources in the PHCT?

Box 2.4   Examples of criteria for deciding the order of priority

The health problem or issue should:

- Be important for the practice population in terms of size (incidence and prevalence) and severity (impact on functioning and clinical parameters)
- Have an existing consensus about its definition
- Be effectively amenable to intervention (including prevention detection and treatment)
- Be feasible for the PHCT
- Attract potential resources to carry out the assessment and to implement any resulting changes
- Be compared with those of external agencies, especially the health authority.

Pitfalls in priority setting

There are a number of potential pitfalls in deciding priorities:

1. No clear criteria agreed or criteria used inconsistently
2. The criteria not being independent of each other
3. Using invalid or complex weighting and scoring systems
4. Having too large a number of options, e.g. 10 or more
5. Trying to rank incomparable options
6. Using rank order as scores
7. Lack of knowledge of appropriateness or effectiveness of intervention
8. Reluctance to make decisions that appear to be 'rationing'
9. Engineering the desired answer by choosing weights that will ensure an option will succeed.

To overcome these difficulties, criteria must be made at the start (each team should modify those suggested here to its own situation). PHCT discussion will usefully clarify the key criteria for that team including new ones.

As HNA involves considerable time in discussion, data gathering and review, then it is important that there are grounds for believing a chosen topic needs improving. Otherwise, as in the example given in Box

---

Box 2.5   Examples

Three PHCTs at an HNA workshop decided the following issues were important for each of them:

- PHCT A: alcohol, asthma, chronic pain, depression, hypertension[*], smoking
- PHCT B: asbestos related ill health, asthma, care of the elderly[*], cervical cancer, ischaemic heart disease, mental health, substance misuse
- PHCT C: alcohol, care of the elderly, child abuse, ischaemic heart disease, management of minor illness[*], reprovision of secondary services in the community.

[*]These issues were decided as the main priority for each team following discussion of the priority criteria for each issue. None was the expected main priority at the start.

2.6, the process can feel useful, but result in little benefit for the PHCT population as a whole.

Box 2.6 Example

A PHCT decided from its practice diagnosis that low birth weight babies were frequent and should be prevented. Having defined low birth weight as under 2.5 kg, the number of such babies was 16 in the past year (25%). The associated risk factors were identified and assessed for each birth; only for two babies were some risk factors not dealt with by the PHCT. The HNA process explicitly clarified why the PHCT thought this was a problem, defined the nature of the problem and what should be done, only to find that the audit showed that little real change could occur as the PHCT were already providing appropriate care.

STEP 4. DEFINE THE EPIDEMIOLOGY – SIZE AND SEVERITY

The problem needs to be clearly defined, otherwise identifying the population which has it will be difficult. Severity is important since a minor problem may not deserve priority. Severity can be difficult to assess precisely, but the key issues to discuss are:

● Does the problem seriously impact on the health status of an individual person or the practice population? Functioning is usefully categorized as physical pain, physical activity, role, and social and mental functioning (Nelson et al 1987)

● Does it present frequently to the PHCT creating a large workload, or rarely but is complex, e.g. upper respiratory tract infection compared to a stroke?

Particularly if a life cycle approach is used (see Ch. 3), then comparison of practice, area, and national demography may be informative.

STEP 5. WHAT SHOULD BE DONE ABOUT THE ISSUE?

If there is little that can be effectively done or changed by the PHCT, then the problem is of low priority for HNA. The evidence for effectiveness and appropriateness of health care needs to be reviewed. Information overload is endemic whether on paper or electronically, so that reviews and summaries of the literature are invaluable but public health advice is useful to develop good critical appraisal techniques (Box 2.7). The local public health department should be able to provide sources of such reviews, whether national, international, regional or local.

Box 2.7 Golden rules for critical appraisal of literature (Sackett et al. 1991)

1. *Title of the article*   Is it relevant to your practice?
2. *List of authors*   Is their track record credible?
3. *Read the summary*   Is the conclusion important to you?
4. *Setting of the work?*   Is it similar to yours to be valid for you in availability of skills, technology and population.

STEP 6. PLANNING
Setting aims and objectives

The whole PHCT needs to understand this simple flow chart of planning:

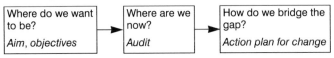

Where do we want to be?	Where are we now?	How do we bridge the gap?
Aim, objectives	*Audit*	*Action plan for change*

Aim is the overall purpose of a programme — what are you trying to achieve? *Objectives* are the specific, desired changes arising from the programme, i.e. the specific outcomes (Box 2.8). Objectives are often muddled with action points, which are how to achieve the desired changes. HNA may also be useful for other purposes such as improving team work or involving other agencies. Objectives that reflect such purposes are called *process objectives* because they are steps in the process of reaching another objective, but at the same time are desirable in their own right. A useful mnemonic for setting objectives is ARMPITS (King's Fund 1994):

Appropriate
Realistic
Measurable
Positive
Important
Time related
Supported by the PHCT

Identifying knowledge, resources and skills

Available information from practice diagnosis needs to be summarized. Any skills gaps need analysis.

Necessary skills

The skills listed below are essential for developing HNA in PHCTs. If the PHCT is missing any of these, that deficiency will soon show as the ideas and challenges of HNA are developed.

1. Team functioning – see check-list for team functioning above
2. Running meetings, timing and keeping minutes

Box 2.8 Example of setting objectives for a PHC diabetic programme

Aim
To minimize the impact of diabetes in the practice population.

Objectives
A. To involve all those patients diagnosed with diabetes in a planned programme of care
B. To ensure all people with diabetes have access to appropriate services
C. To maintain metabolic control of diabetes at a level sufficient to minimize risks of developing complications whilst preserving quality of life
D. To ensure the early identification and treatment of complications.

Action points
1. Identification and registration of all patients with diabetes
2. Full assessment and treatment of newly diagnosed patients
3. Initial stabilization of such patients including educational aspects of the nature and management of diabetes, importance of diet, life-style adjustments for both the person and the carers
4. Maintenance and regular review of metabolic control including well-being and ongoing education
5. Management of acute complications
6. Surveillance for long-term complications and their risk factors
7. Management of long-term complications.

3. Understand planning including objective setting
4. Literature review and critical appraisal
5. Use of libraries and search facilities
6. Be able to keep things simple and not to become side tracked
7. Understand the audit cycle
8. Computer skills:
   – Understand the practice software
   – Know why the PHCT uses a computer
   – Understand Read codes or whatever the system uses
   – Be able to use spreadsheets and word processors.

Resources must be considered very widely:

Resources within the practice Staff knowledge, skills and motivation
Individual patients
Practice budgets
Scope for delegation and creation of available time
Computers

Resources from elsewhere Services available to PHCT
Other PHCTs with experience to share
Health authority, local authority
Academic departments
Voluntary sector
Community groups
External funding

Plan current practice or service review

If carried out, it should identify changes that are needed that the team can make (Box 2.9). But the team may conclude it cannot complete an assessment, or now wishes to do a different one. All these decisions should be a natural consequence of a well-functioning team with common objectives, reacting to collated information.

Box 2.9 Key steps in planning

Aim: overall or global statement of where you want to be
Objectives: desired specific outcomes

● Who is the population involved?
● What are the potential interventions (setting standards) and how effective are they?
● What is being done now for this population and how (relationships between practitioners)?
● What skills, knowledge and resources have we got and what do we need?
● What changes in interventions are needed?
● How is this to be carried out — by whom, when and where, what is feasible?
● What is the important data for evaluation of the impact of the programme?

STEP 7. CHOOSE THE APPROPRIATE METHODS OF ASSESSMENT

Information management (see Ch. 4)

Requirements for data in HNA are to:

● Improve the information for the practice diagnosis to identify priority issues or problems
● Be clear about the size of the priority problem, and which populations it affects
● Know what the determinants of the problem are
● Know what can effectively be done about the problem
● Establish baseline information about what is happening before the programme starts
● Evaluate the process of the programme, i.e. what is actually happening compared with the plan
● Evaluate the outcome, i.e. are the original objectives being achieved?

What data items?

Remember the golden rules of data when thinking about collecting it (Box 2.10). *Data* are items that can be measured, *information* is combinations of data that is useful.

Box 2.10 Golden rules of data

● Be clear about what you need at the start and only collect what you need
● Ensure it is timely, valid, consistent, accurate and complete
● Use available data (e.g. routinely collected for other research) where possible
● Pretest all methods of data collection

Specific issues to consider about data items

1. Most importantly, decide what data are needed and why before collecting them!

2. Is data needed on all the target population? The costs and benefits of collecting missing data must be considered (e.g. is it worth getting 100% of all data about a specific issue, or would 90% do?).

3. Balance the complexity of measures, and the method for collection, against the benefit from those results (e.g. a diet survey is hardly feasible for the whole target population).

4. Methods must be acceptable to the patients (e.g. a diet diary usually is not).

5. Measures, and the collection of data, should form part of mainstream work as far as possible.

6. Are the data items valid (i.e. do they measure what they are supposed to?)?

7. Are data items reliable (i.e. consistent over time or between different people or methods)? Pick items used by good research.

8. Where data are unreliable or unavailable, can estimates be made or is the assessment not possible?

Different data collection methods: advantages and disadvantages

Choosing the right method/tool for data collection is vital, and it is important to understand the most appropriate uses of the various tools for data collection – one method on its own may not be enough. A problem that is associated with all methods is bias, which is systematic errors in the method, giving misleading results. Bias has two main elements:

1. Selection of participants:
  – Definition of disease may be imprecise
  – Survivor-only data miss information from those who died
  – Hospital patients are not representative of those using primary health care
  – A group may have confounding factors, e.g. unemployment
  – Suspicion about key determinants may focus search for disease in an unrepresentative way
  – Nonresponders may be significantly different from the responder group

2. Observer:
  – Recall (inaccurate memory)
  – Interview (his preconceptions motivation may influence responses)
  – Follow-up of drop-outs may be inadequate
  – Misclassification into groups.

Prevention of bias

Selecting population samples. Checking the characteristics of the population you are investigating is important. Does the sample contain the right people for the questions to which the team wants answers? If the respondents are not representative of the population, then it may be difficult to draw true conclusions. In many qualitative studies, a core group of 'key informants' is used who are assumed to be representative of the community as a whole. There may be bias in how individuals obtain positions that permit them to be key informants. Where individuals have different chances of inclusion, false associations and distorted results may occur. Sometimes the only remedy is to be aware of these potential problems in the analysis. At other times a different sampling strategy is used which is deliberately not representative, such as snowball sampling (targeting those who know a lot about the topic) or politically important sampling (targeting those whose support is needed for success) or deviant case sampling (selecting cases from which most learning can be derived). The important lesson here is to avoid generalizing conclusions from unrepresentative data.

Data collection. Specific questions may need designing to avoid bias. Having clear protocols and organizing staff to be appropriately trained is valuable. Triangulation, i.e. multiple methods to reinforce validity, is commonly used

Practical points

Below are a number of practical points that are important when choosing methods:

● What is the availability of resources such as time, skills and equipment? These have to be balanced against the need to use methods correctly. How much experience has the PHCT in using the methods and understanding the strengths and weaknesses of each method?

● What are important data quality issues? Will the method produce information that can be representative of the population, i.e. avoid selection bias?

● Is the method ethical? Can the results be used, or will it raise false expectations, identify previously undetected disease or risk factors for disease?

● Is any relevant information already available elsewhere, and can it be extrapolated to the practice population? Useful sources are the local public health department, the local authority, the CHC and local voluntary groups.

● Is triangulation possible? It is very useful in checking results for consistency and validation. It adds richness to the data from just one method. Many studies use triangulation of three sources of information, and thus 'need' missed by one source will be picked up by another source, rather than need indicated through one source of information perhaps being validated by another source. Therefore, the intended benefit of using three distinct sources of information is lost (Jick 1979, Rossmar & Wilson 1985, Murray & Graham 1995).

Assessment techniques

Chapters 3–11 outline a range of assessment techniques. A summary of the main types is given below.

Qualitative data

Routine data tend to be quantitative (Table 2.2). The retrieval and use of routine practice data are discussed in Chapter 4. The combination of large area routine data and practice data in epidemiologically based needs assessment is discussed in Chapter 6. Questionnaires, interviews and focus groups are techniques which collect quantitative and qualitative data. Qualitative methods strive to attach meaning to human behaviour. They are good for evaluating individualized outcomes, such as getting an overview of programmes where individual patient benefits are crucial, and for finding unusual successes or failures. They are good at describing diversity across programme sites – why and how do local services differ from initial plans and vary across the area. They are used for identifying issues before designing a needs

assessment and for providing a goal free evaluation which eliminates perceptual and evaluator bias from knowledge of existing aims and objectives. They are of course also useful where there is no proven quantitative instrument. But their use requires careful design and often complex analysis. It is crucially important before conducting an interview or questionnaire to seek advice from a social scientist about design. An example found by the London Health Economics Consortium field study from the Mid Essex Health Consortium is:

Q. Do you think worry causes ill health?
A. Yes (in all cases)

What useful information does a question with 100% of responders answering 'yes' produce? A more informative question would be:

Q. Has worry caused you ill health?

This could be useful in showing what people think about the causes of ill health because beliefs affect people's behaviour. Questions that do not identify how behaviour is influenced may not be useful in identifying need, which implies something can be changed. Wherever possible, validated instruments should be used. The long-term illness question in the cases has been shown to be a reasonable proxy measure of disability. Other validated instruments such as SF-36 are too long to allow much room, for other questions (Bowling 1991). They are designed for large populations and may not be valid or provide sufficient detail for small area

Table 2.2 Summary of types of data

Features	Pros	Cons
Routine data collection Data regularly collected often at population sizes much bigger than any one PHCT	Reliable, valid as measures Little effort in collection; often available from other agencies Tends to be reasonably complete	Usually retrospective so how timely is it? For example, the most recent census data is from 1991 Limited in scope May be of limited relevance and insufficiently specific for a particular general practice Causes 'fishing trips', i.e. is used because it is available rather than intrinsically being useful
Collecting specific data from practice records *Record sampling/searches* through practice records or computer database *Patient registers* to identify populations *Audits of guidelines/protocols*: activity and prevalence	Easy to retrieve Can identify groups with clearly definable characteristics	Timely, consistency and accuracy of recording Records what presents to PHCT, and so underestimates prevalence, and is not fully representative of the practice population Completeness may vary, e.g. functional dependency is often missing

studies such as a general practice. Another finding of the above field study was the tendency of interviewers to wish to provide a structure to the interview process. Many failed to avoid the hazard of leading respondents in particular directions, by being insufficiently open. Open questions can be useful to overcome this, but may produce diverse answers which are difficult to classify or interpret, and rely on memory. A compromise might be the use of check-lists which act as prompts for answers (the 'interview guide').

There are two excellent and readable sources of advice – one on qualitative methods generally (Patten 1987) and the other on questionnaire design (Woodward & Chambers 1983) – that should prove invaluable in planning a qualitative assessment of needs. A summary of some of the features of a number of types of technique that involve qualitative methods is provided in Table 2.2. They are further discussed particularly in Chapter 5, Chapter 8 and Chapter 11. Often these techniques are combined in community assessments (see Ch. 11). A summary of rapid appraisal is given in Table 2.4.

STEP 8. WORK IN PARTNERSHIP WITH OTHER AGENCIES

Helpful contacts

- Local health authority primary health care development staff – for team development.
- Local health authority information department – may provide not only information (e.g. courses and activity) but also training on standard computer software packages.
- Local public health department – may provide courses on HNA (such as that run by Judith Hooper, who can provide a course pack).
- King's Fund – King's Fund Community Orientated Primary Care is a complete off the shelf course pack.
- Local postgraduate centre librarian – may be able to help with literature searches.
- Local Medical Audit Advisory Group facilitators – have a wealth of audit packs, literature reviews and some other resources including specific educational courses.

- Local government authority – social services (team managers, lead officer, e.g. disability, elderly, community care plan), housing, and education.
- Local trusts – acute and community trusts (medical director, unit general managers, business plans, quality directorate, current research). Opportunities to work outside the health sector are rewarding (see Ch. 10).
- The Public Health and Primary Care Group – a national group of public health and primary care practitioners which has a database of relevant activities and nationwide membership which could be useful for advice and support. Details are available from Judith Hooper.

STEP 9. SUSTAINABILITY

The key to success is an enthusiastic champion and effective team working. Motivational leadership of the team and the project is crucial.

SUMMARY

Key points to remember and questions to consider:

1. Needs can only exist if something can be done to alleviate the problem
2. Needs always implies a change – will this assessment result in change?
3. Focus on specific areas
4. How well does the PHCT function as a team?
5. Have you defined clearly what you are trying to achieve?
6. For who are you doing the work? Your patients, the PHCT, individuals, the Health Authority?
7. Do the objectives fit the ARMPITS criteria?
8. Are your definitions clear?
9. Are your methods clear and appropriate?
10. Can the HNA be done within existing information, resources and skills?
11. Enthusiastic leadership is crucial.

Good luck! HNA is enjoyable, challenging and very stimulating.

Table 2.3 Summary of qualitative assessment techniques

Features	Pros	Cons
Postal survey, or to patients attending the practice Useful for: ● Prevalence of ill health ● Functional dependency ● Socioeconomic factors ● Knowledge, perceptions ● Use of services in a period of time ● Can link all user perspective activity ● Receipt of advice about specific issues	Time required (minimum) No observer 'bias' Cost low per respondent contacted Quantifiable data/information, assess size of issues Identifies groups that are otherwise difficult to find, e.g. carers Whole practice population available, even those who are remote Requires issues to be identified first, i.e. is a check-list against preset items so useful in audit? Standardized data agreed by practice, enabling compatibility with other surveys using the same questions. Can cover embarrassing or sensitive issues Wide range of issues possible including ill health unknown to the practice	Return rate variable but reasonable from own general practice (65%+) Costs involved for translation Does not identify issues No explanations as to why people think in such a way Representativeness is known Selection bias: ● Young men tend not to respond ● Unilingual questions have limited application ● May exclude the severely disabled, physically and mentally ● Those with damaging health behaviours tend not to respond, especially smokers ● Those with higher educational attainment and social class tend not to respond Actual responder is not known but assumed Complex data collection and interpretation
Focus groups Discussion groups of about 8–15 people; facilitated by a trained moderator and assisted by an observer	Good for exploratory work/or testing theories/concepts Useful for exploring 'why' people think in such a way Useful as a means to backing up quantitative data Good in complex situations or where straight answers are not possible Good for initiating individual views within a group — stimulates debate	Time and costs involved can be high Often criticized as being subjective Training requirements, language and interpreting skills need to be well planned Small numbers of respondents involved Not for use when: ● Respondents are geographically dispersed ● Eliciting the views of the very young or around personal, sensitive issues Lack of rapport with interviewee
Telephone interviews	Cost low Speed of response is quick Ability to target people living in different geographical 'patches', or consult with specific groups of population Useful when simultaneous interviews are required	Interviewer bias Training required to ensure all interviewers use the same approach

Table 2.4 Summary of rapid appraisal procedures

Features	Pros	Cons
Involve key informant interviews, focus groups, and observation of area	Good as a complimentary mechanism for uncovering qualitative issues	Time, coordination
Require the involvement of the practice team.	Relatively quick	Need local practitioners to assist data collection, skills and time – is this possible?
Useful for:	Focused on work 'in the field'	Time commitment required from practice team
● Assessment of health and development needs of community	Semi-structured nature offers flexibility	Only really 'scratches the surface' – no real explanations as to 'why' people say the things they do
● Early stages of project planning	Examine health in a sociocultural context	
● Social relationships and structure	Give richness behind numbers, e.g. perceived predisposing factors for asthma, drug abuse, user views of services	Should not be in isolation – subjectivity
● Culture		Observer and selection bias possible
● Behaviours, attitudes		
● Knowledge, perceptions		
● Defining problems	Allow identification of issues beforehand by the PHCT and during the process from participants, so should be used before a survey	Training requirements
● Assessing strength of feeling on key issues		Requires input from a multidisciplinary team to ensure action
● Identifying resources and solutions, not just problems		
● Eliciting change by just doing it	Participants can partly set the agenda	Wide-ranging needs – too many?
● Identifying characteristics of area		
● Targeting groups or individuals, e.g. PHCT members, carers	Consensus can occur, e.g. priority rating	
	Direct input by key people interview and/or group	

APPENDIX 1. TEAM DEVELOPMENT QUESTIONNAIRE (Woodcock 1989)

Instructions for completion

1. Turn to the answer grid at the end of this questionnaire
2. Work through the statements, in numerical order and put a cross in the appropriate square of the grid if you think a statement about your team is broadly true. If you think a statement is not broadly true, leave the square blank
3. Do not spend a great deal of time considering each statement; a few seconds should be long enough
4. Remember that the results will be worthwhile only if you are truthful

'Building blocks' questionnaire

1. Our team lacks leadership
2. Decisions seem to be forced upon us
3. People are not encouraged to speak out
4. When the going gets tough it is every one for herself, or himself
5. Communication needs improving
6. Decisions are taken at the wrong level
7. Some of the managers are not true to themselves
8. We seldom question the content or usefulness of our meetings
9. Insufficient development opportunities are created
10. We are frequently at loggerheads with other departments/organizations
11. Team members do not communicate with each other sufficiently
12. The accepted order is rarely challenged
13. No-one is really clear where we are going
14. People do not say what they really think
15. People have an 'I'm all right Jack' attitude
16. Conflict is destructive in this team
17. There is inadequate information on which to base decisions
18. Some of the managers are not trusted
19. We do not learn from our mistakes
20. Managers/senior team members do not help their subordinates to learn
21. Relationships with other groups are 'cool'

22. We do not project our position well within the organization and our constituency
23. We often find that we lack the required expertise
24. We are all very busy but we do not seem to get anywhere
25. Issues are brushed under the carpet
26. It would help if people were more willing to admit their mistakes
27. There is mistrust and hostility
28. People are uncommitted to decisions
29. There is little team loyalty
30. Outside opinions are unwelcome
31. There should be more job rotation
32. We seldom work effectively with other teams
33. We fail to secure cooperation from other teams or departments
34. No-one builds the necessary bridges with other groups
35. We do not spend adequate time planning for the future
36. Delicate issues are avoided
37. People get 'stabbed in the back'
38. We do not really work together
39. Inappropriate people make the decisions
40. Managers are weak and not prepared to stand up and be counted
41. I do not receive sufficient feedback
42. The wrong kinds of skills are developed
43. Help is not forthcoming from other parts of the organization
44. There is a great deal of misunderstanding between our team and the other interest groups who impact upon us
45. We do not pay sufficient attention to relationships
46. We do not have a clear view of what is expected of us
47. Honesty is not a feature of our team
48. I do not feel strengthened by my colleagues
49. Skills and information are not shared sufficiently
50. It is the wrong personalities that get their own way
51. Dignity is not recognized
52. We should spend more time questioning the way we operate
53. Managers do not take personal development seriously
54. The rest of the organization does not understand us
55. We fail to get our message over to the outside world
56. We often reach decisions far too quickly
57. The way an individual is valued has little to do with what is achieved
58. There are too many secrets
59. Conflicts are avoided

60. Disagreements fester
61. Commitment to decision is low
62. Our manager(s) believe(s) that tighter supervision improves results
63. There are too many taboos in this team
64. There are manifestly better opportunities in other departments
65. We put a lot of energy into defending our boundaries
66. Team members do not understand what is expected of them
67. We do not pay sufficient attention to new ideas
68. Priorities are unclear
69. People are not involved sufficiently in decision-making
70. There are too many recriminations
71. There is not enough listening
72. We do not utilize the skills we have available
73. Managers believe that people are inherently lazy
74. We spend too much time doing and not enough thinking
75. Individuals are not encouraged to grow
76. We do not try to understand the views of other teams
77. We fail to listen to our customers
78. We tend to move before reaching conclusions
79. We do not understand what other departments are aiming at
80. Some people back down too easily
81. Generally there is low trust here
82. People are unwilling to take the views of others into account
83. We do not consider alternative solutions sufficiently
84. Yesterday's attitudes prevail with our manager(s)
85. The accepted order is rarely changed
86. Our manager(s) lack(s) the skills to develop others
87. We have too little influence on the rest of the organization
88. We could really use some training on how to improve communications
89. We have too many specialists in our team
90. Managers do not plan for the future together
91. In this team it pays to keep your mouth shut
92. A lot of time is spent 'defining' territory
93. There are too many fights
94. People feel frustrated because they are not consulted
95. Management does not care whether people are happy in their work
96. We seldom change our working procedures or organization
97. We should spend more time developing our own senior people
98. We do not reach out to help other groups
99. The left hand doesn't know what the right hand is doing
100. We are not sufficiently results orientated
101. Different parts of the organization are pulling in different directions
102. People are not prepared to put their true beliefs forward
103. People are not really helped to develop
104. This place reminds me of a battlefield sometimes
105. There is a need for more democracy
106. Managers take little action to make employees' jobs interesting and meaningful
107. Delicate issues are not raised
108. Many people trained by the organization later join other organizations
109. Ideas from outside the team are not used
110. We lack the information we need to do the job
111. We pay too little attention to the quality of our work
112. Our aims are not democratically agreed
113. Team members do not get sufficient honest feedback
114. People should stand on their own feet more
115. We should discuss our differences more
116. Team members are not sufficiently involved in taking decisions
117. Our leader(s) does/do not make the best use of us
118. We should seriously consider the relevance of our meetings
119. Individual development is stifled by the team
120. Information does not flow freely enough between teams
121. Good ideas do not reach those who could implement them
122. We have too many people with similar skills
123. We should place more emphasis on results
124. People 'hear what they want to hear' rather than the truth
125. More time should be devoted to discussing fundamental values
126. We do not get down to the root of our differences

127. Decisions are taken at the wrong level
128. Our leader is not true to his own beliefs
129. We should take more account of how others see us
130. People are discouraged from being authentic
131. The organization as a whole is not a happy place to work in
132. There is too little 'listening'

Building blocks' answer sheet

Follow the instructions given at the beginning of the questionnaire. In the grid there are 132 squares, each one numbered to correspond to a question. Fill in the top line first, working from left to right; then fill in the second and subsequent lines. Be careful not to miss a question.

A	B	C	D	E	F	G	H	I	J	K
1	2	3	4	5	6	7	8	9	10	11
12	13	14	15	16	17	18	19	20	21	22
23	24	25	26	27	28	29	30	31	32	33
34	35	36	37	38	39	40	41	42	43	44
45	46	47	48	49	50	51	52	53	54	55
56	57	58	59	60	61	62	63	64	65	66
67	68	69	70	71	72	73	74	75	76	77
78	79	80	81	82	83	84	85	86	87	88
89	90	91	92	93	94	95	96	97	98	99
100	101	102	103	104	105	106	107	108	109	110
111	112	113	114	115	116	117	118	119	120	121
122	123	124	125	126	127	128	129	130	131	132

Totals

When you have considered all 132 statements, total the number of crosses in each vertical column and write the score for each column here. This is your score for

A	Balanced roles
B	Clear objectives and agreed goals
C	Openness and confrontation
D	Support and trust
E	Cooperation and conflict
F	Sound procedures
G	Appropriate leadership
H	Regular review
I	Individual development
J	Sound intergroup relations
K	Good communications

REFERENCES

Adelaide Medical Centre Primary Health Care Team 1991 A primary health care manifesto. British Journal of General Practice 41: 31–33

Bowling A 1991 Measuring health. A review of quality of life measurement scales. Open University Press, Milton Keynes

Jick T J 1979 Mixing qualitative and quantitative methods – triangulation in action. Administrative Science Quarterly 24: 602–611

King's Fund 1994 Community-orientated primary care. King's Fund, London

Murray S M, Graham L 1995 Practice based health needs assessment: use of four methods in a small neighbourhood. British Medical Journal 310: 1443–1448

Nelson E, Wasson J, Kirk J et al 1987 Assessment of function in routine clinical practice – description of the COOP chart method and preliminary findings. Journal of Chronic Disease 40 (Suppl 1): 55S–63S

Ong B, Humphries G, Annett H, Rifkin S B 1991 Rapid appraisal in an urban setting. An example from the developed world. Social Science and Medicine 32: 909–915

Patten M Q 1987 How to use qualitative methods in evaluation. Sage, London

Rossmar G B, Wilson B L 1985 Numbers and words – combining quantitative and qualitative methods in a large scale evaluation study. Evaluation Reviews 9: 527–543

Sackett D, Haynes R B, Guyatt G H, Tugwell P 1991 Clinical epidemiology. Little, Brown, London

The Royal College of Nursing 1993 The GP practice population profile. Royal College of Nursing, London

Woodcock M 1989 Team development manual. Gower, London

Woodward C, Chambers L 1983 Guide to questionnaire construction and writing. Canadian Public Health Association

Techniques of assessment

3

The life cycle framework

Ian Williamson   Chrissie Pickin

Chapter 2 highlighted the criteria for successful health needs assessment and the criticality of choice of issues and of populations. The requirements seem quite daunting. This chapter seeks to show a simple practical way of approaching needs assessment for the busy general practice which has never done it before. It draws on qualitative information, rather than using statistics. The model of the Life Cycle Framework can be helpful in working through problems and in devising solutions.

First, the aim of general practice health needs assessment (GPHNA) should be agreed: 'to support those making decisions by providing information about health problems, possible options and solutions, which will enable a practice to improve the health of their population'. GPHNA can then be seen as a way of making more rational decisions. Underlying this is the key issue of motivation. Those working in general practice should ask themselves the following question: *'Do we want to change the ways we practice and make decisions?'*

Before starting any GPHNA, the practice would benefit from exploring the following questions:

1. *Are we able to change our current ways of working? Are we willing to do things differently?* (Box 3.1)

For example, are you able to change the referrals you make to secondary care if the needs of your practice population and evidence of effectiveness suggest that you should? Would you be willing to do so and risk upsetting a secondary care colleague? Are you willing to change your prescribing patterns if other, more appropriate, drugs or treatment methods seem to be more

---

Box 3.1   Case study

One practice team in Salford met at the start of a health needs assessment project. They were facilitated by the family health service authority and a local research centre, and the whole team (including attached community staff) decided that it could change its ways of working with the aim of improving the health of the practice population.

effective for certain conditions? Are you willing to try new ways of treating patients, both within the practice and in partnership with others such as community nursing or social services? This may mean changing the staffing within your practice – employing a psychologist, a physiotherapist, a counsellor or a chiropractor. Are you able and willing to make these decisions – either alone or in partnership with your local health authority?

Responding to health needs assessment means change to you and your practice. If you are happy with the status quo, practice-based health needs assessment is not worth the time, energy and effort involved.

2. *Are we willing to make decisions about the way in which we work?* (Box 3.2)

Box 3.2 Case study

Representatives from several general practices, together with other health, social services and youth workers in the same locality, built up an enthusiasm to change, and a project was set up to improve the lives of older people and young men in the area.

The ability to change working practices in primary care is dependent upon team working, as a practice's internal resources are so interdependent. One of the prerequisites for being able to implement the action plans of any health needs assessment is that the 'team' can truly function as a team and support the necessary change. So, a key question you need to ask is: 'Are we a team or just a group of individuals?'

Unless there is some clarity about who is in your team and what roles each of you have, the results of needs assessment will be very hard to implement. One result of general practice health needs assessment may be better team working, but this requires good leadership and genuine commitment from all parties. So choosing needs assessment as an enjoyable and interesting way of improving teamwork is an option. This may help practices explore the way for them to respond most appropriately to the primary care-led National Health Service (NHS) policy. But if this is your aim, start simple.

3. *What can we make decisions about?* (Box 3.3)

Do you feel that all the important decisions about health services in your district are made by people you never see and don't know and that your views are rarely taken into account? While these feelings are still commonplace

---

Box 3.3 Case study

Massive reductions in waiting times for ophthalmology, from up to 2 years to a standard of 2 weeks, resulted from pressure from general practitioners which was fed to the health authority through a series of face-to-face interviews held between them and health authority directors.

---

in primary care, there are examples (and not all from fundholders) where general practice has made a real difference. Our work in Salford and Trafford has involved general practitioners (GPs) successfully making improvements in ophthalmology waiting times by changing referral patterns and working with the health authority to provide primary care-based eye clinics. Others across the country have made significant input into major service changes by working in partnership with their local health authority. Although your practice team can only make decisions directly for itself, you can work in partnership with your local health authority or GP multifund or locality commissioning group, to make major secondary care service changes. Any health needs assessment methodology therefore needs to be able to promote change in both primary and secondary care. You need to know what decisions you are making daily that influence the health of your practice population and what decisions your local health authority is making that you can influence for the benefit of your patients.

GPHNA should not be seen only as a way of allocating development or growth money. The majority of resources for health in any practice are within its own team members. GPHNA is as much about changing the way in which team members work as it is about changing referrals and influencing secondary care professionals.

Box 3.4 summarizes the questions that GPs should ask themselves before undertaking health needs assessment.

Box 3.4 Key questions to consider before starting GPHNA

- Are we able to change our current ways of working?
- Are we willing to do things differently?
- Are we willing to make decisions about the ways in which we work?
- Are we a team or just a group of individuals?
- What can we make decisions about?

CHOOSING THE POPULATION SUBGROUP AND PROBLEM AREA TO FOCUS ON (THROUGH THE LIFE CYCLE FRAMEWORK)

Exploring the above areas is likely to highlight a number of organizational issues which you and your practice will want to tackle. Some of these (e.g. holding team meetings, taking team decisions and sticking to them) may not directly impact on the health of the practice population but must be worked through if you are to reap the full rewards of health needs assessment.

Having commenced this, you are now ready to address some of the health problems in your practice on a population basis. The practice population is so large and diverse and the needs are so great that it is important to target your health needs assessment work. Many methodologies for health needs assessment start from a service perspective and target on services where there are problems with access, e.g. long waiting times, or with quality, e.g. where operations are cancelled, discharge letters are delayed or where there are concerns about clinical effectiveness. We believe that this service-led approach leads to a focus on secondary care solutions and as such does not take advantage of the many other resources for health that exist within primary care. We therefore feel it is important to use a population subgroup as the way to focus the work. The 'life cycle framework' offers a way of supporting this approach. This approach is explained further in the book *Assessing Health Need Using the Life Cycle Framework* (Pickin & St Leger 1993).

The life cycle framework divides the population to be studied into nine life stages from before birth to old age (Box 3.5). From the age of 15 years onwards the life stages are also subdivided by gender, because after this age the health experience of women is significantly different to that of men.

Its value is that it takes into account the biological, psychological and social determinants of health. The life stages are chosen because they represent periods in people's lives when certain factors tend to predominate in determining their health experience. Thus the health of a woman between the ages of 25 and 44 years is likely to be influenced by her fertility and be related very much to child bearing and child rearing. Men's health between the ages of 15 and 24 years is likely to be determined by their developing sexuality and their changing image of themselves as adults, and consequently there is an increasing likelihood of involving themselves in unhealthy behaviours.

Box 3.5   The nine life cycle stages

1. Late pregnancy to 1 week after birth
2. 1 week to 1 year
3. 1 year to 4 years
4. 5 years to 14 years
5. 15 years to 24 years
6. 25 years to 44 years
7. 45 years to 64 years
8. 65 years to 74 years
9. Over 74 years

Dividing the practice population into groups of people in life stages takes into account the importance of age and gender in determining its health experience. Age and gender are of course not the only influences on health. The framework therefore introduces 'modifiers'. These are factors known to influence the health experience of a population over and above that caused by age and gender. They are classified under four headings:

1. Socioeconomic
2. Environmental
3. Ethnic
4. Cultural

In Pickin & St Leger's book, the nature and extent of likely modifiers to health are identified and explained for each life stage. Thus the framework allows for a health status profile to be drawn for each of the life stages. Each life stage profile can then be used for health needs assessment by relating each life stage to local service provision or policy development.

Advantages of a life cycle framework

The advantage of the life cycle framework over other ways of identifying health need is that as a general approach it fits with the scientific and intuitive understanding of the determinants of ill health. More specifically:

1. It forces detailed examination of the needs of differing groups of people in a coherent way.
2. It encourages you to look at what information you require to make decisions about this population group and does not force thinking to be constrained by what information is currently available.
3. It provides a framework which can link information, planning and resource allocation in a more coherent way.
4. It allows health influences to be related to service provision, either current or proposed, health service or non-health service, curative or preventative, and not just to secondary care services.
5. It explains rather than just describes the health of a population, and is therefore educative.
6. It easily accommodates an increase in our knowledge of the determinants of health and health service utilization in a population.

Suppose that you and your team decided that you wanted to look at the possibility of assessing the health needs of young children (from 1 to 4 years of age) in your practice (Box 3.6). You would first want to look at the major causes of death, illness and disability in this population group. Death is very rare in this age group but those that do occur are largely due to congenital abnormalities or accidents and violence. Do you know all the children on your list with major congenital abnormalities? Do you know what their major health problems are – from your perspective and their parents'? Are their needs for developmental surveillance, therapy services, play, education, respite and palliative care being met? Children of this age tend to experience more home accidents than road traffic accidents. Are your health visitors aware of problems in your practice population with home safety? Do they have a programme to improve parents' understanding of and access to home safety? Does the practice team have a clear policy about non-accidental injury?

The major cause of morbidity in this age group is diseases of the respiratory system. Although many of these are mild and self-limiting they are exacerbated by parental smoking and damp housing conditions. Do you have children on your list with recurrent respiratory

Box 3.6 The life cycle framework – a worked example. The health of young children aged 1–4 years

1. What population group do we want to explore the needs of in more detail?	Children aged 1–4
2. What are the major causes of death, disability and abnormalities, and illness in this group?	Deaths – accidents, violence, congenital Disability – behavioural disorders Illness – respiratory problems, etc
Choose an area to explore	Respiratory problems
3. Appropriateness a. Are you offering the most appropriate service?	Ask parents their needs
b. Are you seeing all the children with respiratory problems who would benefit from seeing a PHCT member?	Use prevalence figures from the local health authority to predict numbers expected and compare with your practice morbidity data
c. Are there problems with any relevant 'modifiers' in your local community?	High proportion of parents smoking? Poor quality damp housing on local estate? Main road with standing traffic near local school causing air pollution?
d. Can you identify an organization which can help reduce the level of modifiers?	Highways agency? Housing department?
4. Effectiveness Are you offering the most effective practice?	a. What are you trying to achieve? b. What do effectiveness bulletins say about this issue? c. What other evidence of effectiveness do you know, e.g. prescribing, investigations, referrals? d. To agree with PHCT the most appropriate and effective practice for this client group e. Audit local practice against these standards f. Produce practice guidelines on management of URTI in young children
5. Efficiency Can you use PHCT staff in a different way to achieve the same outcome at a lower cost? Can you prescribe more cheaply and achieve the same outcome? Can you manage or refer differently and achieve the same outcome at a lower cost?	Brainstorm ideas within the PHCT and discuss with the local health authority, e.g. pharmaceutical advisers

prescribing policy for this group? Do you follow a period of 'watchful waiting' before referral to an ENT surgeon for those with glue ear? Have you examined other forms of treatment for glue ear, e.g. homeopathy?

Asthma is a major cause of morbidity in this age group. Do you have an asthma register? Do you know how many children you would expect to have asthma in your practice population? How many are you aware of? Why don't you know about the others? What are their health problems – from your perspective and the parents'? Do you have a treatment protocol agreed by the practice team? Are you clear when to refer on? Are these based on the latest research evidence?

The commonest cause of disability in this age group is behavioural disorder. How many of your practice's children have a major behavioural disorder? Do you provide parent training within the practice? Do you have clear guidelines for referral to clinical psychology services? Do such services exist in your area? Would your practice population have difficulty accessing the services that are available – because of poor bus routes for example?

Using the life cycle framework and asking questions such as those posed above will enable you to draw up an overview of the health problems and service issues that need to be addressed both within the practice team and outside. This overview is essential should you wish to carry on with detailed health needs assessment work in order to improve the health of this particular section of the practice population.

CLARIFYING WHAT YOU ARE TRYING TO ACHIEVE

Having decided on a particular subgroup of your practice population and having identified the key health issues that you wish to focus on – for example, childhood asthma (Box 3.7) – you can then focus even more by clarifying what you are trying to achieve in relation to relevance to need, effectiveness and efficiency. Essentially the aim of health needs assessment is to maximize all of these, yet there is often a trade off between them. In looking at any health problem within the practice it will help to be clear which is the most dominant issue: relevance to need, effectiveness, efficiency or cost containment. The following definitions may be helpful.

Relevance to population need

This is the extent to which the service meets the needs of a group or a population for which the service is intended. In planning terms it is the population which is the relevant denominator, and thus its relevance to needs is: 'the extent to which the service(s) meet the needs of the whole population with those problems'.

For example, is the service the practice offers in terms

disease? Do they live in poor housing conditions? Are they from a particular locality or estate? Can you discuss the problems with your local social services department or with the local housing department? Are they entitled to all the benefits they should be receiving? Can any of your team members do anything to encourage their parents not to smoke in the house (or at all)? Do you have a of practising and referral appropriate to the needs of children with asthma – will it meet all of the needs of all the children with asthma under your care? Are there difficulties in some schools with enabling children with asthma to take what is prescribed? Are some children unnecessarily missing school? Is hospital referral the best way of dealing with this?

This is a key issue when there is substantial unmet need in a hidden population. For children with asthma this is likely to be the case. It is also important when the health problems likely to be experienced are many and diverse and there has been a tendency to look at just immediate medical needs. In the case of children with asthma are there any emotional needs of the parents and children that need to be met? What are they?

Effectiveness

This concept can be limited to an individual or to users of a particular service, or can extend to the whole population. Effectiveness is 'the extent to which the service delivers the desired results'.

Public health specialists use the term to refer explicitly to beneficial changes in health of people, causally related to the service. Managers more commonly use it in its broader sense to refer to whether the service changed anything.

In order to say whether something is effective or not we need to know what it is trying to achieve, i.e. effective at what?

In this case we would limit our approach to just those children with asthma that we know about. We would decide what exactly we were trying to achieve, e.g. fewer deaths, reduced hospital admissions, less time off work for parents, reduced complications, improved forced expiratory volume, or reduced anxiety among

parents, and we would then look at whether these can be measured and find the practice that is most effective in producing our desired aim.

Another example is the aim 'to reduce teenage pregnancies' – is the service we offer effective at doing this?

Efficiency

Efficiency is 'the extent to which the service delivers the desired results at the lowest cost'.

Economists talk of 'technical efficiency' – the various mixed staff, supplies and equipment to get a given output, and 'economic efficiency', and which is the lowest cost combination to do so. The latter is the key one that focuses attention on cost minimization, using the lowest grade of appropriate staff.

Using the example of asthma again, if efficiency is the most important issue, we would ask which of the effective services was the most cost-effective. Could we achieve the same results with a lower cost drug or delivery system? Could we reduce referrals to a hospital-based clinic by employing our own asthma nurse and running practice-based clinics for our population and others in the locality?

As another example, if our aim is to get people with acute back pain back to work as soon as possible, we need to know which is most efficient – referring to a chiropractor or to the orthopaedic outpatient department.

Cost containment

This is limiting activity to fit a given amount of money. It does not have a focus on results or needs.

For example, my prescribing budget is overspending – how can I reduce it?

CHOOSING THE TYPE OF HEALTH NEEDS ASSESSMENT REQUIRED

Having chosen a population group, identified the key health and social issues using the life cycle framework and the key outcome issues regarding relevance to need, effectiveness and efficiency, we can now look at what form of health needs assessment will be required to develop an action plan. We have worked with four different ways of relating services to health problems. Each has advantages and disadvantages at both the health authority and practice levels.

Population-based health needs assessment

The first is population-based health needs assessment. This follows most obviously from the life cycle framework approach to health problems in that it starts from the population health needs. It is therefore the only type of health needs assessment that comprehensively looks at the issue of relevance to need. It will also provide evidence on effectiveness and efficiency and so allows trade-offs between the three outcomes. An example is given in Box 3.8.

There are three key elements to the process.

1. Provision of sufficient, relevant information

Such information is needed on:

a. *Health problems*, from three perspectives – epidemiological, professional and lay.

The epidemiological perspective gives information on the impact of that particular health problem on the population as a whole. It will also give a picture of trends over time. Epidemiological information is information on mortality, morbidity and disability. Much is routinely available at a district level but needs to be disaggregated to practice level. This may lead to problems with too small numbers for analysis. However, this should not stop you getting a general feel for the important health issues within your practice. Spending some time looking at 'the bigger picture' is a stimulating way of reflecting on the way individual practitioners use their time, and may highlight areas where need and demand diverge.

The professional perspective on problems gives depth and detail to the epidemiological perspective. Views from local experts can be very useful in identifying health problems, but professional orthodoxy can restrict the view. The professional perspective is available by talking to colleagues and reading the professional literature.

The lay perspective gives detail from the patients' perspective or their carers. It will give insight into the impact of the health problem on an individual's life. It is a more holistic picture but is restricted to views based on the current situation. This makes it less useful for long-term planning purposes, particularly with large population groups, but at the practice level it can provide very illuminating information.

In view of the fact that this approach is looking at relevance to need, we need to get this information on all those with the particular health problem of interest. The epidemiological view will give some indication of unmet need, the professional view rarely does and it is the lay view of those not currently using services that provides such a rich source of information to develop relevant services. This information is difficult to get and needs to be obtained through research. Increasingly, market research methodologies are being used in social research to get these types of views, and these lend themselves to work within primary care. An example is focus groups where a trained researcher carries out a group interview with, for example, a group of parents of young children with asthma.

b. *Health resources*. Resources for health are more than just money. They include:

- Resources within an individual, e.g. motivation
- Resources within a family, e.g. family income and availability of social support
- Resources within the community, e.g. baby-sitting circles and church groups
- Resources within primary care
- Resources within secondary care
- Resources within tertiary care
- Resources within the local authority services, e.g. meals on wheels, day care, respite care, and nursing home care
- Resources within the voluntary and independent sector.

Having obtained a clear and comprehensive picture of the problems, it is important to identify a comprehensive view of the resources on offer within your practice population to help them address this health problem. For example, for children with asthma, is there a local self-help group, are there families able to offer support? For those with disabilities what resources exist within the local community?

Whether you have direct influence over them or whether they involve money or not, it is important to be aware of all health resources, as some real beneficial change can occur simply by advertising existing resources, or by changing current practice slightly, e.g. opening times.

c. *Health outcomes*. Clarifying exactly what you are trying to achieve in health terms is important at this stage. Is your main priority to reduce deaths, reduce morbidity or improve quality of life – and in which areas? Only having clarified this can you look at the literature on effectiveness.

Box 3.8 Case study. Alcohol health needs assessment with general practice

By supporting a health authority-led health needs assessment exercise, general practice helped to ensure that an alcohol strategy was developed and implemented. The result was alcohol specialist staff based in practices, working with GPs and practice nurses to identify and address many of the problems alcohol causes.

All three perspectives on alcohol need identified that under-age drinking, binge drinking and their consequences were major issues – yet virtually no resources were directed to them. It was agreed that the desired outcomes would focus on resolving these problems.

When options were discussed, it was clear that action had to be taken jointly with other agencies, but also that effective, brief interventions in primary care would be appropriate.

The action taken included investing in primary care alcohol workers, paid for out of disinvestment from some inpatient services, and healthy alliances to work towards reducing alcohol-related street violence.

2. Development and appraisal of options

Up to this stage we have been looking at health problems rather that looking at solutions. It is important to suspend looking at solutions too early as our professional orthodoxy tends to detract us from developing innovative, effective interventions if we think of solutions too early. But now having a clear and comprehensive view of the problems, potential health resources in our community and a clear sense of what we are trying to achieve, we can begin to generate solutions.

Try to come up with at least 10 ideas covering preventive care, treatment and supportive care. Brainstorming is a useful way of approaching this.

Having identified as many possible options to address the health problems and achieve our desired outcomes then we may need to appraise them using explicit criteria. The type of criteria we have used within primary care to appraise options are:

- Meet the needs identified from all perspectives
- Have evidence of effectiveness with this population group from research literature
- Have evidence of effectiveness from practice elsewhere
- Most cost-effective option
- Consistent with the values of the organization
- Consistent with lay values.

Using these criteria we then prioritize the list of options to meet the need. This should lead to a list of cost-effective options that are relevant to need. From this you can outline the optimum ('ideal') service.

3. Development of an action plan

We frequently speak to people frustrated by the lack of quick action which results from their health needs assessment. We respond in two ways: firstly, that health needs assessment will indeed take longer than just deciding to 'do something', and, secondly, that we try to avoid such frustrations by having and implementing a clear action plan.

The action plan sets out the optimal service from preventive care, through treatment to support. It then sets out the steps to be taken by the practice to move from the current position to the optimal one. It also includes areas of other's practice that if changed could be beneficial for your patients – this gives you an agenda for discussion with the local health authority, social services, local voluntary sector groups, local patients groups, etc. We have found it helpful to write action plans under four headings, as shown in Box 3.9.

The aim and process of population-based health needs assessment are summarized in Box 3.10.

Box 3.9 An action plan

a. What do I need to invest extra in – more time, energy, staff, money?
b. What current ways of working do I and the team need to carry out differently?
c. What do I need to do less of to free up time, money, staff and energy to accomplish step (a)?
d. What could others do differently that would help me to carry out my action plan or otherwise improve the health of this group?

Box 3.10 The process of population-based health needs assessment

Aim: to support those making decisions by providing information about health problems, possible options and solutions which will enable a practice to improve the health of their population.
Elements:
1. Provides sufficient, relevant information on health problems, resources and desired outcomes
2. Generates and appraises options to meet the identified needs
3. Development of an action plan which is clear what has to be done, by when, by whom and in what way.

Other forms of health needs assessment

All other forms of health needs assessment that we recommend are variants of population-based approach (Box 3.11). The second type is service based, or health *care* needs assessment. This limits identification of health problems to those experienced by current and potential users of *existing* health services and the available resources for health to current health and social care. It assumes that services are generally relevant to need and therefore the agenda is to improve access, effectiveness or efficiency. The process is as described above except that we do not need to research the health problems of those who may require a service that does not as yet

---

Box 3.11 Other types of health needs assessment – a summary

Health care needs assessment
- Limits identification of health problems to users of existing services only
- Could be used to address the needs of, for example, insulin-dependent diabetics.

Fast track needs assessment
- Only a local action plan is new, other work is copied from elsewhere
- Could be used around coronary heart disease in two neighbouring localities.

Service review
- Concentrates mostly on efficiency-based changes to services
- Could be used to follow-up population health needs assessment that was done a few years' previously, i.e. where there is confidence that the service is now relevant to need and effective.

exist in a mainstream way. This means that the research is much less time-consuming and the option generation takes a narrower focus. The downside is that we can miss major health problems. For example, a service-based approach to eye care would look at the needs for ophthalmology services and would concentrate on exploring effective and efficient solutions to meeting the needs of people with cataracts, glaucoma, trauma and diabetic retinopathy. It would, however, miss the needs of people with age-related maculopathy – the most prevalent condition causing visual disability in older people. The population-based approach would have identified this as a major problem and would have identified options to meet the need, e.g. rehabilitation officers to develop skills which will improve sufferers' quality of life. If unmet need is not thought to be a particular problem and the population in need is the same as the current or potential users of existing services, e.g. insulin-dependent diabetics, then this approach is as valuable as the population-based approach. It is just as good at identifying effective and efficient solutions and is quicker than the population-based approach as the research is less time-consuming. It may be an important first step for general practice needs assessment.

Another variant is what we call 'fast track needs assessment'. This is a short cut by adapting other people's work to your population. Its validity increases with the similarity of the two populations. Where it is assumed that the two populations are sufficiently similar or the differences are known and the effects on needs are qualified it is useful to borrow others' needs identification or option generation work. The third step of developing an action plan still needs to be done. Some local ownership may be lost through not using local data, but the process is much faster.

A fourth variant is not really health needs assessment at all. It is the familiar service review. This does not explore the needs of the population or service users in any great depth, nor does it address issues of effectiveness in any great detail. A service review generally looks at the way an existing service is delivered to see whether changes can be made to reduce the cost or increase the effectiveness of care. However, the process assumes that the current need for services and the desired results have not changed. It is therefore most useful when cost containment or efficiency is the prime requirement.

CONCLUSION

Health needs assessment at a primary care level is more than developing practice profiles or health needs identification. The assessment part of it requires a sophisticated and systematic approach to generating and appraising options and developing an action plan for change as a result. Health needs assessment is of use in building teams in general practice, but its real value is as a decision-making tool to develop services that appropriately, effectively and efficiently address the health problems in a population. The nature of primary care practice makes it eminently suitable to identify health problems but its loose and often individualistic nature makes the later stages of option generation and appraisal and action plan development much more difficult. This is the challenge for practice-based health needs assessment. The life cycle framework and our experiences in Salford and Trafford have helped us produce a few mental maps along the way. We hope you find them useful.

REFERENCE

Pickin C, St Leger S 1993 Assessing health need using the Life Cycle Framework. Oxford University Press, Oxford

4

Using routine practice data

John Shanks   Sadru Kheraj

This chapter illustrates some of the applications of information which are readily obtainable by most practices. Some of the information will already be available within the practice itself, some is easily extracted from the local health authority, other types may require that practice staff have previously collected it.

Some of the information is *quantitative* and expressed in numerical form (e.g. numbers and age mix of registered patients); some is *qualitative* (priorities and preferences of patients expressed in a satisfaction survey).

The common aim behind all the applications is to produce better quality decisions – by the practice, by prospective patients, and by health authority managers concerned with allocating resources (Shanks et al 1995). Chapter 12 will focus more on the methodological and technical issues involved in the use of this data. Chapters 5 and 8–11 look at qualitative measures and the different types of qualitative data which are readily obtainable. This chapter concentrates on standard quantitative data.

Most of the examples given here refer to general practice, but it is possible to apply similar information to other primary care services such as community pharmacy or health visiting.

This chapter mainly uses the practice population as a convenient unit of analysis. Many primary care services are delivered and organized at the level of single practice populations, and it is an easily identifiable unit. But sometimes it is more appropriate to consider a larger unit of population such as a local authority borough – for example, in relation to social services or community care. Or it may be useful to group several practice populations together where they form a commissioning group, a multifund or a locality.

WHY BOTHER?

Table 4.1 shows some of the uses which practice-based information can serve for three different groups of interested people.

Table 4.1 Uses of practice-based information by various groups of people

Practice staff	Health agency managers	Patients
Clinical audit	Interpreting audit results	Select a suitable practice
Plan practice development	Plan developments	Inform response to consultation
Bid for new resources	Allocating resources	Lobby for client group or disease
Forecast future demands	Prioritizing bids from practices	

EXAMPLES

Age–sex registers

An age–sex register is basically just a list of the practice population which includes information on patients' age and gender. Registers of this type were developed initially in the 1960s (Pinsett 1968). They can be a valuable basis for planning services because the likelihood of many different types of health problem is partly determined by age or gender. In the past, there have been doubts about the completeness and accuracy of practice age–sex registers (Sheldon et al 1984) but increasing direct electronic linkage between the practice and the main age–sex register at the DHA should make it easier in future to maintain up to date records (Brazier 1994).

Practice profiles

A practice profile is just a convenient, often graphical, summary of key information about the practice and the population it serves. It usually includes basic data such as that contained in the age–sex register together with other information relevant to health and health services such as data from the census analysed down to the small area level (Crayford et al 1995). Even if the information is already familiar to members of the practice, bringing it together in one place in an accessible format allows it to be used by a wider audience and compared to other practices, and may highlight previously unnoticed features.

Figures 4.1–4.4 show for four different practices in south-east London a few key pieces of information assembled in graphical format and compared to local averages:

1. The age–sex structure of the registered practice population compared both to the catchment area from which the practice draws its patients and to the whole DHA area
2. The social characteristics of the community in the practice catchment area
3. Some measures of activity in the areas of prescribing, cervical screening and patients leaving the practice without changing address

Lambeth, Southwark and Lewisham Health Authority produce for each practice a standard format profile containing these items with a guide to interpretation.

Hospital referrals

Variations in the use of hospital resources are of great interest too, because of the large resource costs involved. It is usually impossible to say what would be the 'best' rate of referral for any condition, but practices may wish to review their referral behaviour from time to time, particularly if it is unusually high or low compared to others or following a change in service which might be expected to make a difference, e.g. a new practice policy on the management of asthma.

Some sort of comparison helps to make sense of the referral rate for a practice. This could be the referral rates for either other practices in the same commissioning area, the same small locality or some other chosen group such as other practices of similar size and type. Or it may be possible to compare the practice with itself at different points in time, looking for changes or trends.

Figure 4.5 shows an extract from a regular newsletter sent to practices in Camden and Islington Health Authority. Each newsletter is individualized so that the practice to which it is addressed can see how it compares to other local practices (Scobie et al 1995).

Clinical activity – prescribing, health promotion, and practice annual reports

A practice may wish to know how it compares in terms of the activities, services and treatments it provides. This could include such things as family planning, minor surgery, child health surveillance, health promotion and home visits. There are special fees for many of these, and so detailed financial records have to be collected by the DHA in order to make the appropriate payments to practices. This financial information can be reused to measure the level of activity of the practice in any service for which there is a special payment. As with hospital referrals, there is usually no 'correct' or 'best' level. Comparison with other practices or at different points in time allows the practice to identify where there may be scope to increase activity in a particular area, thus generating more income, or reduce activity and divert resources elsewhere. So a practice might identify that its level of claims for family planning services is low compared to other practices of similar type but that there seem to be plenty of young adults on the list who might wish to make use of such services if the practice developed and advertised these. Conversely, the practice may identify that it has an unusually high rate of claims for home visits and decide that it would like to save some of the professional time which these visits represent for use in another, possibly more constructive way.

Prescribing

Prescribing data have a dual value. Firstly, they provide information about one rather important clinical activity. Secondly, they can act as a proxy marker for the health problems which certain drugs are used to treat – the prescription of insulin, for example, acts as a marker for the prevalence of insulin-dependent diabetes.

Prescribing data are derived from returns made by the PPA (Prescription Pricing Authority) and analysed centrally as Prescribing Analysis and Cost (PACT) data. The PACT system was set up in 1988, initially to provide general practitioners with information about prescribing costs (Prescription Pricing Authority 1995). The system has since been extended, and every general practitioner now receives quarterly information about prescribing. The level 3 reports produced by the PPA contain a catalogue of all the prescriptions issued by a practitioner for the previous quarter and contain a range of useful analytical information. PACT data is based on prescribing units, and so indicates how much of a particular drug a practice prescribed but not how that quantity was divided among patients. It cannot therefore distinguish between the effect of a few patients receiving very large quantities of a drug or many patients receiving smaller prescriptions of the same drug. Practices which use their own computers to produce prescription forms will generate, as a by-product of this, information on the pattern of prescribing which can be related to individual patients or groups of patients to fill in some of the gaps from PACT data. Fundholding practices may find it particularly useful to examine prescribing, since it has proven to be an area in which large savings can often be released quite readily by increasing the rate of generic prescribing or reviewing the use of high-cost drugs. Non-fundholding practices may be eligible for incentive payments for reaching identified targets for generic prescribing rates, for example.

It is possible to examine issues of clinical effectiveness and good practice through prescribing data: the ratio of inhaled steroids to bronchodilators prescribed is now commonly used as a measure of how effectively asthma is being managed. In general, a higher ratio indicates better management, and so a practice or a group of practices can include the steroid:bronchodilator ratio within an audit of asthma management and look for improvement over time (Fig. 4.6). Conversely, high levels of prescribing of specific drugs of 'limited therapeutic value' such as appetite suppressants or benzodiazepines may indicate a practice which is experiencing or creating problems.

With patient-centred prescribing information from the practice computer it may be possible to identify patterns of prescribing which the practice would like to change. Figure 4.7 shows for one practice the age distribution of patients who are receiving long-term prescriptions for benzodiazepines. The practice was considering a campaign to offer support for withdrawal or reduction for long-term benzodiazepines users. The information here suggests that there may be two different groups of patients: a younger group with a median age of about 35 years and an older group with a median age of about 65 years. These two groups may require different approaches and different types of support to withdraw successfully.

Health promotion

The Wycombe Primary Care Prevention Project has been running since 1986 with a focus on developing the effectiveness of health promotion and chronic disease management in South Buckinghamshire (Tapsfield 1995). As part of this, the project publishes a regular newsletter and works with individual practices to help them develop methods of population-based needs assessment.

The Health Education Authority operates a national database for health promotion in primary care.* The database can provide information on specific local health promotion initiatives in primary care and also details of courses and training available.

One practice in a deprived community piloted a new patient registration questionnaire with the objective of testing an opportunistic approach to case finding and health promotion (Fig. 4.8). A total of 1290 questionnaires were satisfactorily completed with a 90% response rate; largely due to the simple 'yes/no' design. A practice algorithm guided action to positive answers. For example, those respondents answering positively to night cough or wheeze were considered to be potential asthmatics, and offered an appointment and clinical assessment. Those children who admitted to not being able to swim, or those elderly who admitted to hearing loss, were sent leaflets about appropriate classes or services. The impact of the project was to improve recording of preventive care data in records, establishment of the profile of cardiovascular risk factors in the registering population, which was particularly high, and refocus clinical practice for coronary risk patients onto facilitating fitness and exercise provision, which was clearly demanded. If this technique were extended to more representative samples of general practice populations, it could form the basis of a comparative needs assessment with national norms in areas in which morbidity and risk factor prevalence data are not normally available – such as incontinence, hearing loss and alcohol abuse.

*Telephone: 01685 225587; Fax: 01865 741980

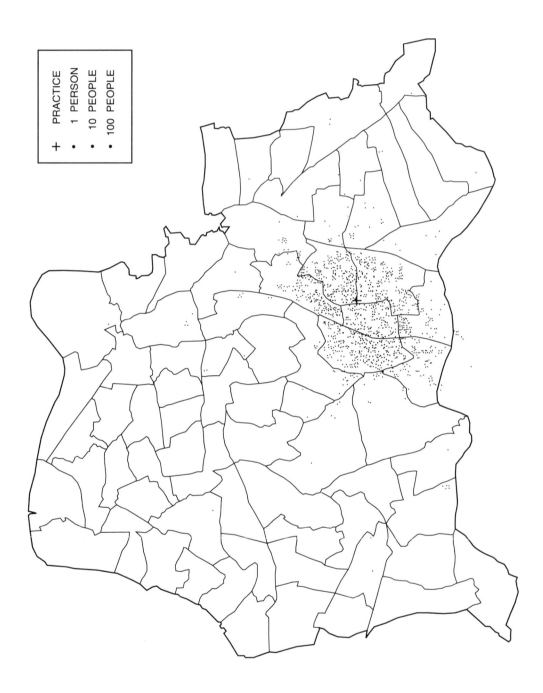

Figure 4.1 The geographical distribution of registered patients for two practices in south-east London. The boundaries are electoral wards. This knowledge is important when considering locality needs assessment where the degree of coterminosity between practice and geographic boundaries is critical (see Ch. 8). **a** This practice has a relatively large list size with a very compact distribution around the practice premises. **b** This practice has a much smaller list size which is thinly scattered over a much larger area.

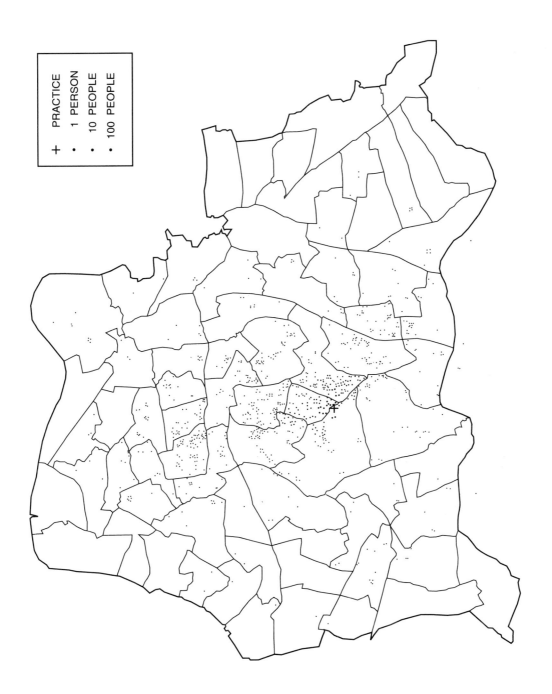

(b)

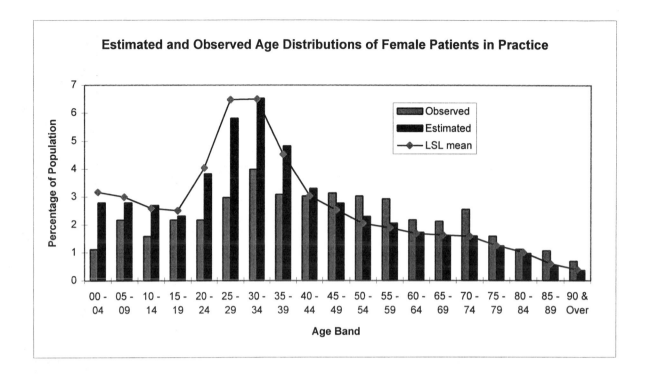

(a)

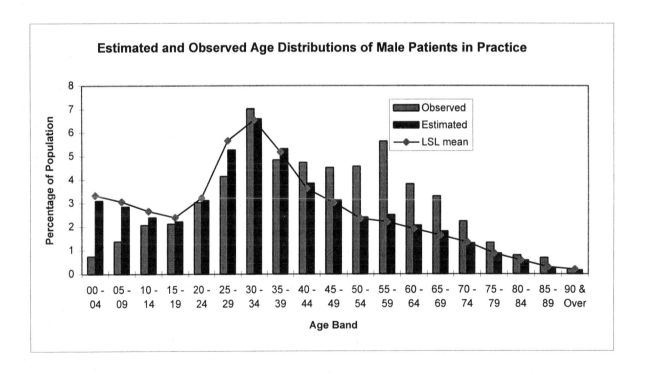

(b)

Figure 4.2 The age–sex distribution for the registered list of a single-handed male practitioner in south-east London (Lambeth, Southwark and Lewisham Health Authority) who has practised from the same premises for many years. **a** Female patients. **b** Male patients. Note the relative deficit of young women and children and the preponderance of elderly people on the list. 'Observed' is the actual mix of registered patients; 'estimated' is what would be expected from the composition of the population in the practice's catchment area; 'LSL mean' is the average for the whole FHSA area.

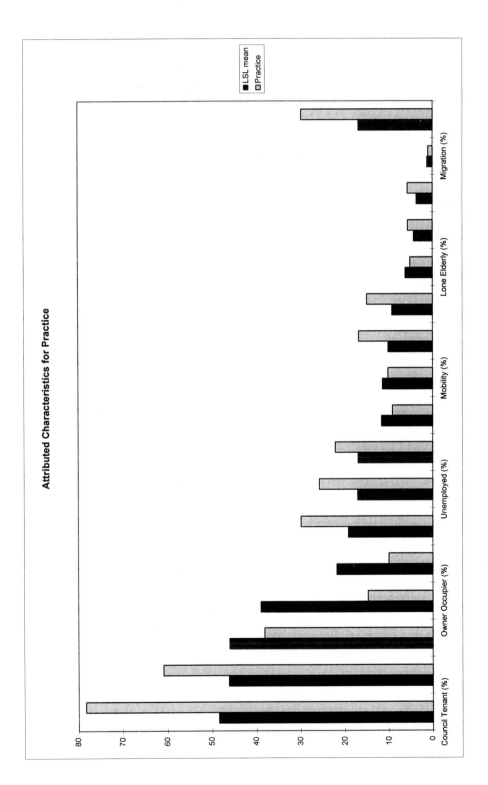

Attributed Characteristics for Practice

Figure 4.3 Attributed social characteristics of a practice population. This gives an estimate of the social characteristics which the list of registered patients would be expected to have if they are typical of the catchment area from which the practice draws its patients. For each characteristic, the predicted value for the practice population is compared to the average value for the DHA (Lambeth, Southwark and Lewisham Health Authority) area as a whole ('LSL mean'). These predicted values are derived from the answers which local people in this area of south-east London gave to the most recent national census in 1991. The practice shown here has a higher than average Jarman score, which means it is serving a more than usually deprived population. The prediction is for higher than average proportions of people who are from ethnic minority groups, lone parents, council tenants, without access to a car or living in overcrowded accommodation. Knowledge of the size of the practice list (the denominator) and the prevalence of the measured characteristic in the population are needed to judge the significance of variations from the norm. Small practices and rare attributes increase the likelihood that variations are not significant.

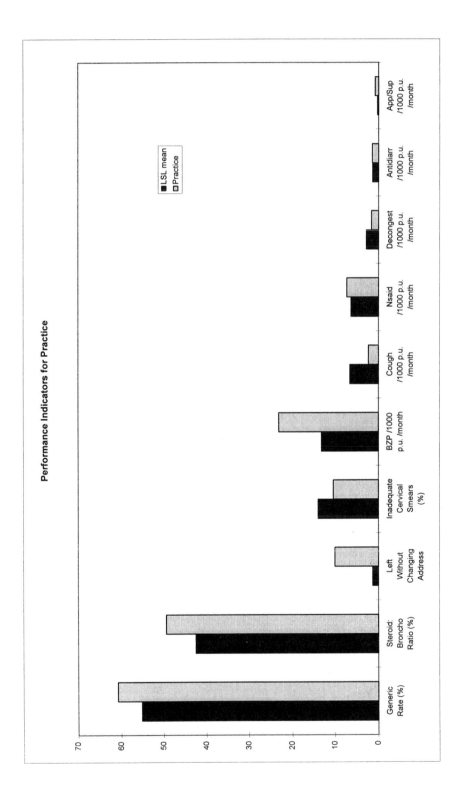

Figure 4.4   A set of indicators which can be obtained readily from routine data on prescribing, patient registration and cervical screening. These may help to throw some light on areas of practice activity which are going particularly well or which merit review. The value for the practice is compared in each case to the average value for the DHA (Lambeth, Southwark and Lewisham Health Authority) area as a whole ('LSL mean'). The two indicators on the left of the area are conventional markers of good prescribing: in simple terms, the higher these values are, the better. The other eight indicators are ones where a lower value is usually better: the proportion of cervical smears which are returned as inadequate, the proportion of patients who leave the practice without changing address, and the prescribing rate for a selection of drugs of 'limited therapeutic value' such as benzodiazepines, cough and appetite suppressants, systemic decongestants, antidiarrhoeals and topical non-steroidal anti-inflammatory agents. For the practice examined here, most of the values are better than the local average with the exception of benzodiazepine prescribing, which seems rather high. The practice used this information to review its benzodiazepine prescribing policy.

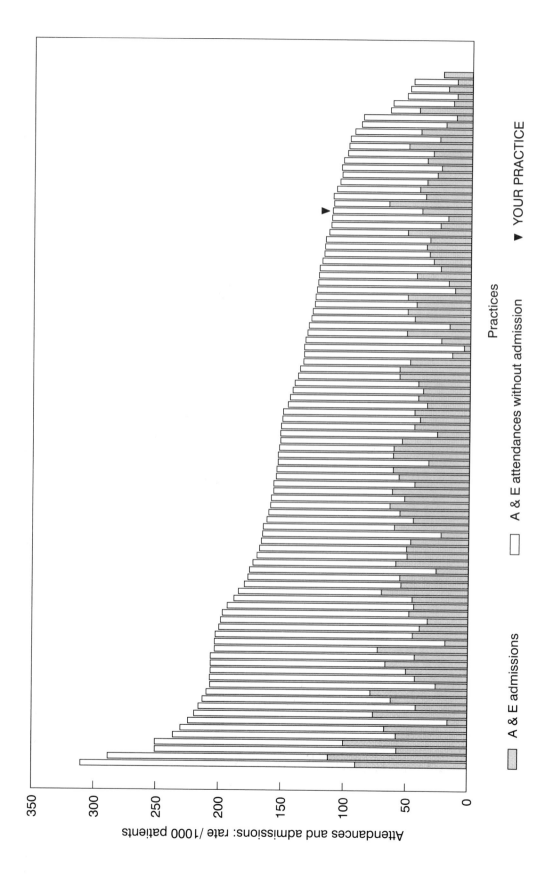

Figure 4.5   The rates of patients attending and being admitted from accident and emergency departments for all practices in the Camden and Islington area of north London. A very high level of accident and emergency referrals, particularly if few seem to lead to admission, might indicate that some patients are self-referring or being referred with the sort of urgent problems which could potentially be managed within primary care. (Reproduced, with permission, from Scobie et al (1995).)

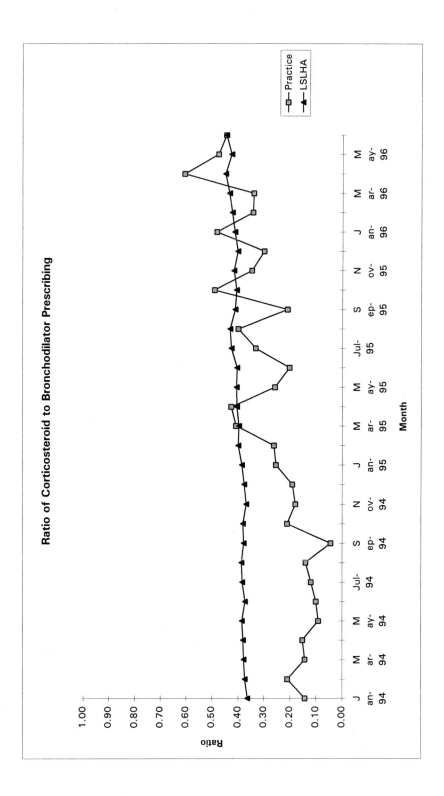

Figure 4.6   How the steroid : bronchodilator ratio altered over a period of time for one practice in south-east London which changed hands from an elderly single-handed practitioner to a group of younger practitioners during this interval. ■, practice; □, DHA average.

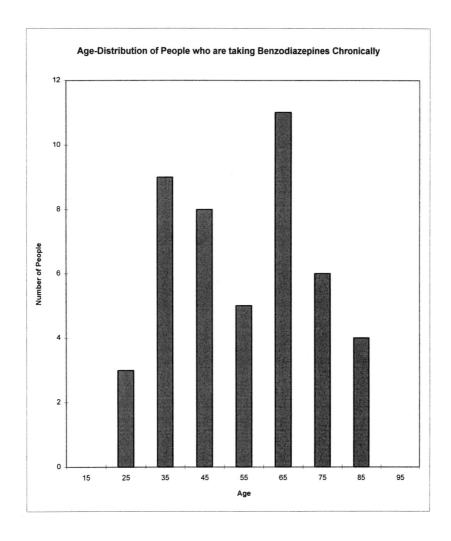

Figure 4.7   The age distribution of patients receiving long-term prescriptions for benzodiazepines from a practice in south-east London. (Reproduced by kind permission of Dr Tim Crayford.)

The practice annual report

Although the production of an annual report is sometimes viewed as an unwelcome externally imposed task, a recent survey showed that many practices would continue to produce one even if not required to do so because of its value to the practice itself (Record et al 1994). South Staffordshire Health Authority plans to use information derived from the practice's own annual report as part of a health needs assessment pack provided to the practice (Iqbal & Walsworth-Bell 1995).

Morbidity – patient records and disease registers

It can be very useful to get a picture of the sort of health problems presenting to a practice in order to identify where it might be possible to improve the match between services on offer and what patients require. This might involve introducing a new service to meet an emerging demand.

The individual patient record is the most obvious source of information about health problems. The traditional 'Lloyd George' style patient note does not generally lend itself easily to systematic data extraction or analysis, although John Fry was able to use a written system to collect and analyse information about consultations in his practice over several decades (Fry 1979). The widespread adoption of computer systems that record clinical consultations, and the introduction of standard coding systems such as Read to classify encounters, mean that high-quality data about clinical activity can be readily obtained. At present, this sort of information is only patchily available. In 1993, it was estimated that 71% of practices had computers that could record clinical consultations (NHS Management Executive 1994). Questions still remain about the quality and consistency of this data (Mant & Tullock 1987, Gilliand et al 1992). Increased collaboration between practices may help to improve this. In Wakefield and Pontefract, 14 practices collaborated to share computerized information about coronary heart disease risk factors, diabetes and asthma and to assess the need for community-based rheumatology services (Wilson et al 1995). Further research into present information use and its role in managerial decision making will help assess the impact of information exchange.

The Royal College of General Practitioners conducts periodic national surveys of the pattern of problems presenting to a sample of practices across the country (Royal College of General Practitioners et al 1995). This gives an average national picture. Things may be very different at a local level, but it may be possible to make use of the national information by identifying and making allowance for the ways in which a particular practice is known to differ from the national average, e.g. by having an older or younger age mix of registered patients. Ideally, a practice would find it most useful to have access to information on the sort of health problems experienced by its own patients. Some of the information necessary to get such an individual picture would have to be specially collected, but some may be available from more routine sources such as chronic disease management clinics or health promotion activity.

A practice which operates a chronic disease management programme for asthma or diabetes, for example, will have information on the number of known diabetics or asthmatics, the type of treatment they are receiving, and perhaps some outcomes from regular reviews of these patients. For most other conditions, the practice must look to information which it has itself collected during consultations or by means of occasional special surveys of registered patients or the local community.

Figure 4.9 shows information retrieved from diagnostic data held on a practice's own computer. The diagnosis shown here is hypertension. There are many ways in which such information can be used, for example:

● To provide an estimate of the total number of patients affected, allowing predictions to be made on the likely number of staff and other resources required to run a service such as a regular hypertensive review clinic.
● To provide a baseline against which to compare the profile of subgroups from the hypertensive population, e.g. the age–sex profile of patients attending for their regular blood pressure check may show that younger men are under-represented and may require some special initiative to contact them.

Note that for this practice the rate of diagnosed hypertension is higher for women than for men at all ages. This is a detection phenomenon. In reality, hypertension is more common in men, but general practice offers many more opportunities to detect hypertension in women – in the course of family planning or antenatal visits, for example. There is probably a deficit of undiagnosed hypertension among men in the practice. If the practice decides to set up a well man clinic or some other special initiative to pick up hypertension in men, then one measure of the success of this could be to check if the male–female gap narrows in later versions of this display.

There are some limitations inherent in this practice-collected morbidity data. This information can only illustrate problems which patients actually consult about and which are recognized by the practice. It inevitably misses out on those health problems which affect people not registered with a practice (e.g. homeless people) or which patients do not consult about or which the practice does not pick up (e.g. unrecognized depression or other psychological problems). The biggest problem is inconsistency or incompleteness of the data. If the general practitioner or other practice staff only fill in the diagnostic data on some patients, then the picture will be a partial and distorted one. If different general practitioners or different practices have different and unspecified concepts of, for example, hypertension, then it makes it difficult to compare or interpret figures on the numbers of people with untreated hypertension.

Mortality

For most individual practices, the number of deaths which occur over the course of a year is too small to allow any meaningful analysis. It may be possible, particularly for larger practices, to aggregate deaths over a number of years to produce a 5 year average, for example. This might allow a practice to look at trends in mortality from some of the bigger causes of death, such as heart disease. Computerized practices may be able to retrieve their own information on deaths. Other practices could request the local health authority to analyse from their records of all deaths in the district those which occurred among patients of the practice. It may be easier to make sense of mortality data for a defined geographical patch of a number of practices in a small locality.

Resources allocated to the practice – practice staffing and community nursing

Practices and DHAs often want to examine the level and type of resources in a practice to check that the practice is getting a fair share and to identify gaps where additional input may be required. This exercise may be more

GENERAL NEW PATIENT REGISTRATION QUESTIONNAIRE   LEAVE BLANK

Answering these questions will help the doctor plan your care.   No.
The information will be treated confidentially.

NAME   DATE OF BIRTH   Age 16–59

DATE OF REGISTRATION . . . .

Are you in any way disabled   PLEASE TICK
making it difficult for you to: CORRECT ANSWER

Get to the surgery?	NO . . .	YES . . .	1
Use the public transport?	NO . . .	YES . . .	2
Use the telephone?	NO . . .	YES . . .	3
Read letters?	NO . . .	YES . . .	4

Are you concerned about your:

Weight?	NO . . .	YES . . .	5
Fitness?	NO . . .	YES . . .	6
Smoking?	NO . . .	YES . . .	7
Alcohol consumption?	NO . . .	YES . . .	8
Stress?	NO . . .	YES . . .	9
Have you ever had high blood pressure?	NO . . .	YES . . .	10

Does your mother, father, sister, brother have
angina; or have they ever had a heart attack
or stroke?   NO . . .   YES . . .   11

Have you ever been thought diabetic?   NO . . .   YES . . .   12

Have you ever had chest pain from your heart,
or a dizzy spell, thought to be a mini stroke
or actual stroke?   NO . . .   YES . . .   13

Do you ever cough in bed at night or on running?   NO . . .   YES . . .   14

Have you ever wheezed?   NO . . .   YES . . .   15

Have you any previous problems of a
psychiatric nature?   NO . . .   YES . . .   16

Are you looking after an elderly, frail
or disabled relative living with you?   NO . . .   YES . . .   17

Are you currently attending hospital?   NO . . .   YES . . .   66

Have you ever felt bad or guilty about your
drinking?   NO . . .   YES . . .   69

Have you ever had a drink first thing in the
morning to steady your nerves?   NO . . .   YES . . .   70

Notes

NR Appt.

Action

EXTRA QUESTIONS FOR WOMEN OVER

EXTRA QUESTIONS FOR WOMEN   LEAVE BLANK

At what age did you first take
the oral contraceptive pill?   Never . . .   After 20 . . .   16–20 . . .   18
                                                                            Before 16   19

When did you last have a cervical
smear test?   Date . . . .   Within 3 years   Never . . .   20
                                            More than 3 years ago . . .   21

Have you ever had a hysterectomy?   NO . . .   YES . . .   22

How many miscarriages or abortions
have you had?   None . . .   One . . .   22
                                                            More than one . . .   23

What age did you have your first child? 20–30 . . .   Under 20 . . .   24
                                                                 Over 30 . . .   25

Has your mother or a sister had
breast lumps removed?   NO . . .   YES . . .   26

When did you have a breast check?   Within 3 years   More than 3 years ago   27
                                        Date . . . .   Never . . .   28

Have you had any vaginal bleeding
or discharge since the menopause
("Change")?   NO . . .   YES . . .   29

Have you children aged under 5 years?   NO . . .   YES . . .   30

Are you ever depressed?   Rarely . . .   Sometimes . . .   31
                                                                 Often . . .   32

                                                                            Notes

                                                                            WW Appt.

                                                                            Action

Figure 4.8   A new patient registration questionnaire as devised by one practice. (Reproduced by kind permission of Dr Andrew Harris.)

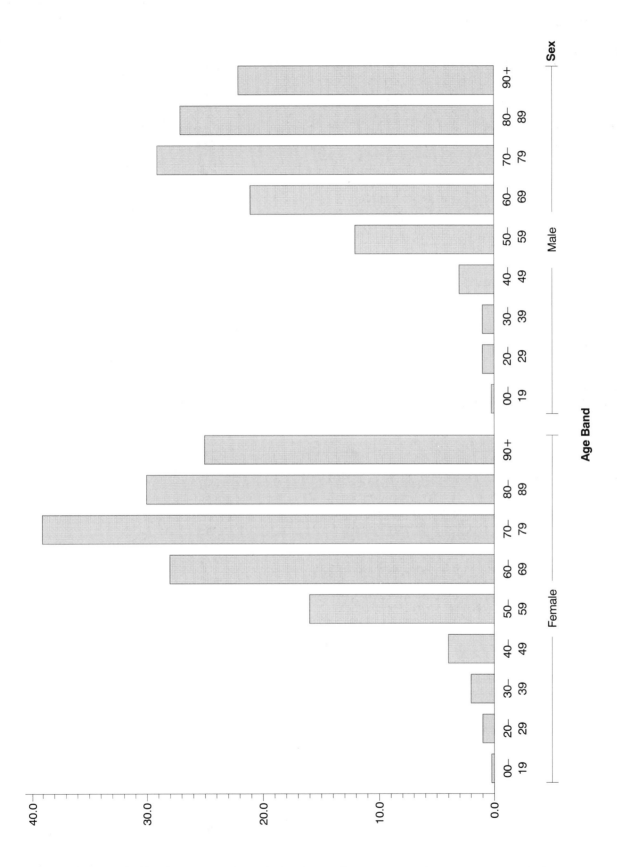

Figure 4.9   The age and sex distribution of patients who have been diagnosed hypertensive and are receiving antihypertensive medication for one practice in south-east London. (Reproduced by kind permission of Dr Tim Crayford.)

useful if it can be set alongside information about the practice population or clinical activity. It is possible to represent the level of allocation of various types of practice staff compared to the number of registered patients.

Table 4.2 shows for one DHA area in south-east London (Lambeth, Southwark and Lewisham) how the distribution of various types of practice staff compares to the national average. In a similar way, an individual practice can compare its own staffing allocations against local and national averages. This sort of comparison may identify practices which have historically had much lower levels of resources than others but which appear to be serving populations with high levels of need for primary health care. A practice in this position might use such information to strengthen a bid for additional resources, an DHA with limited additional resources for practice staffing might use the information to identify those practices which should have priority on the basis of need. Resource allocation to localities is discussed in Chapter 8.

Depending on the particular type of health need under consideration, it may be sensible to look at one particular staff group, e.g. if a practice population has been assessed as having a probably higher than average need for mental health care on the basis of high deprivation and high unemployment rates, then it would be sensible to see how that practice population compares to others in terms of allocation of mental health specialist staff resources such as counsellors and clinical psychologists.

Similar calculations can be made in respect of community nursing staff employed by local community health trusts and attached to the practice.

Primary health care services beyond general practice

Similar considerations and methods can be applied to other primary health care services such as dentistry, community pharmacy or optometry.

A DHA is responsible for the whole range of primary health care services and will want to take a needs-based approach across the board. A practice may also be interested in assessing the requirement for pharmacy or dentistry services because of the impact which these services (or the lack of them) can have upon the patients of the practice and demands made on the practice's own services. It seems likely that pharmacists, for example, will increasingly work as part of the primary care team (Ford & Jones 1995, Barber et al 1994).

Some of the same sorts of information are available as for general practice in respect of specific services for which there is a payment, but in general there is less detailed information on patients who use the service.

Table 4.2 Distribution of practice staffing resources by staff type comparing England and Wales to Lambeth, Southwark and Lewisham (LSL) in south-east London.

(a) Core practice staff employed by general practitioners

Total practice staff	England and Wales	LSL
No.	84 700	522
Whole time equivalent (WTE)	54 019	853

	England and Wales		LSL	
Practice staff type	WTE	Percentage	WTE	Percentage
Total	54 019	100	853	100
Practice manager	6 498	12	109	13
Computer operator	1 315	2	41	5
Secretarial/receptionist	34 475	64	541	63
Dispenser	1 000	2	–	–
Nurse	9 640	18	157	18
Other/unknown	1 092	2	5	1

(b) Percentage of general practitioners offering various services[a]

	Minor surgery	CHS	Maternity medical services	Contraceptive services	Health promotion programmes[b]		
					Band 3	Diabetes	Asthma
England and Wales	76	93	96	100	91	89	89
South East Thames	75	94	93	99	90	88	90
LSL	48	55	96	85	75	77	79

[a]LSL data: *MIS*, April 1993. England and Wales, and South East Thames data: *NHSME – GMS Medical Statistics*, October 1992.
[b]Source: Oracle; percentages calculated by No. of practices in each band and multiplied by the No. of general practitioners in each practice.

Community pharmacy

Figure 4.10 looks at the geographical distribution of one type of special service provided by some community pharmacists in south-east London – needle exchange for injecting drug misusers. It would be desirable to ensure that pharmacies in areas where drug misuse is most prevalent offer needle exchange services. Local data on the location of drug misuse can be hard to find, but there are some possible proxy markers which may guide decision making. It has been shown that in an inner city area, the unemployment rate is quite closely correlated with the prevalence of illicit drug misuse (Squires et al 1995). Therefore, mapping unemployment rates (derived from the National Census or other surveys) gives a guide to where illicit drug misuse is likely to be concentrated and, therefore, where needle exchange services might be most usefully located. Although some of the pharmacies offering needle exchange seem to be well located relative to likely drug misuse, there are areas of expected high drug misuse where there is no pharmacy offering needle exchange and some pharmacies which do offer the service appear to be located away from where drug misuse is most prevalent.

Community ophthalmic services

Optometrists are offering an increasingly wide range of primary eye care provision, including services previously provided only by medical practitioners such as screening for diabetic eye disease (Logie & Haines 1995, Ryder 1995). To maximize the benefit to health, these services need to be planned on the basis of information about the local population who are the potential users. As with community pharmacy services, this might include using population characteristics as proxy markers of health

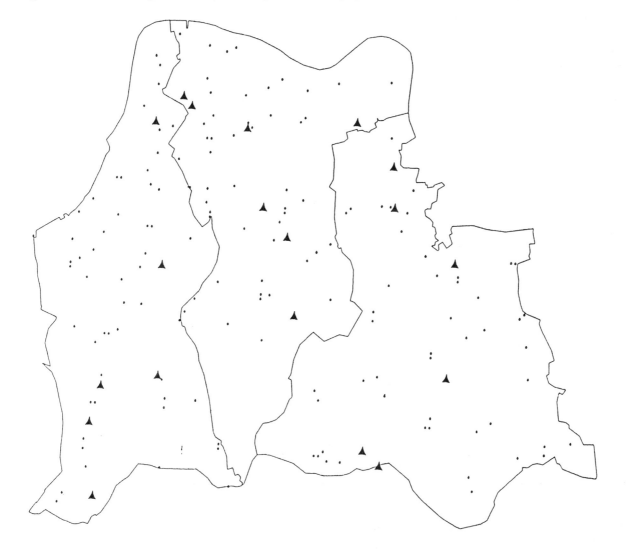

Figure 4.10   Pharmacists in Lambeth, Southwark and Lewisham who offer a needle exchange scheme for injecting drug misusers. A triangle indicates a pharmacy offering needle exchange. Other pharmacies are indicated by dots. (Source: Oracle, September 1995; Information Directorate.)

need to predict where particular services are most needed. For example, an area with a high proportion of elderly people or people of Indian, Pakistani or Caribbean origin is one where good availability of diabetic eye screening would be particularly important.

Community nursing

The level of district nursing and health visiting services available to a practice is directly relevant to the ability of the practice to provide services to young children and older people and the workload placed on other members of the practice team. It is very important for a practice to ensure that the allocation of community nursing resources is appropriate to its requirements and used to best advantage.

A practice which wanted to review its use of community nursing resources might start off by considering how it is placed relative to other local practices. Figure 4.11 shows an attempt to do this for district nursing allocation to practices in south-east London. What one might hope to see is that practices serving similarly deprived populations would have a similar allocation of district nurses for a standard number of elderly people and that there would be a tendency for more deprived practice populations to receive a larger allocation of district nursing than less deprived ones. The actual picture

looks very different from this; practices of similar levels of deprivation were found to have quite different levels of allocation of district nursing, and some of the most deprived practice populations have some of the lowest allocations of district nursing time. This tends to confirm the impression that there are some inequities in the current distribution of resources.

These profiles may be a useful starting point for collaborative work with community trusts (see Ch. 9). Indeed, much routine practice data are just that – it is the skill in analysis and imagination in usage that generates the needs assessment.

CONCLUSION

In conclusion there is a wealth of available data, but practitioners and managers alike may benefit from training and advice about their appropriate usage. At present it is largely being used as a health profiling exercise, but some comparative needs assessment is generating questions about existing provision and practice. There is a need to evaluate more closely the impacts of the exchange of data and information. This can be facilitated by greater explicitness about our decision making processes and information needs.

DISTRICT NURSE SKILL-MIX ADJUSTED ALLOCATION

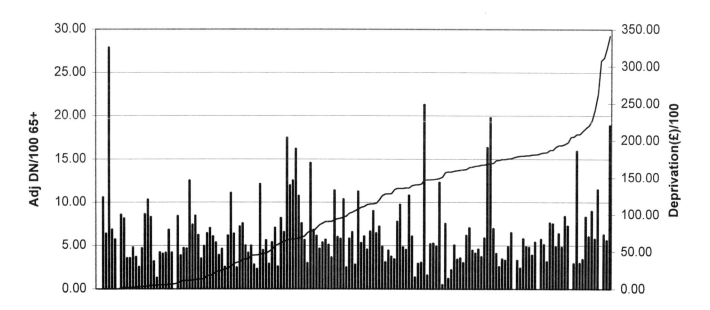

Figure 4.11 Allocation of district nursing staff time to practices in Lambeth, Southwark and Lewisham, showing whole time equivalent (WTE) district nurses per 100 registered patients aged over 65 years. The chart shows on the left-hand vertical axis for each of 170 or so practices the number of WTE district nurses allocated to the practice for every 100 patients over the age of 65 years on the practice list (average = 0.41). Practices are ranked from left to right in ascending order of deprivation as measured by the proportion of patients on the list who attract deprivation payments. The wandering line shows on the right-hand vertical axis the percentage of the practice population which attracts deprivation payments. (Sources: Oracle, January 1995; WLCCT, April 1994; Information Directorate.)

REFERENCES

Barber N, Smith F, Anderson S 1994 Improving the quality of health care: the role of pharmacists. Quality in Health Care 3: 153–158

Brazier W 1994 List matching. Lambeth, Southwark and Lewisham Health Commission, London

Crayford T, Shanks J, Bajekal M, Langford S 1995 Analysis from inner London of deprivation payments based on enumeration districts rather than wards. British Medical Journal 311: 787–788

Ford S, Jones K 1995 Integrating pharmacy fully into the primary care team. British Medical Journal 310: 1620–1621

Fry J 1979 Common diseases. Croom Helm, London

Gilliand A E W, Mills K A, Steele K 1992 General practitioner records on computer – handle with care. Family Practice 9: 441–450

Iqbal Z, Walsworth-Bell J, Wardle S 1995 Healthcare needs assessment in primary care. A pilot project. Department of Public Health, South Staffordshire Health Authority, Stafford

Logie D, Haines A 1995 How can we improve the detection of glaucoma? British Medical Journal 310: 546–547

Mant D, Tullock A 1987 Completeness of chronic disease registration in general practice. British Medical Journal 294: 244–247

NHS Management Executive 1994 Computerisation in general practice – 1993 survey. Department of Health, London

Pinsett R J F H 1968 The evolving age–sex register. Journal of the Royal College of General Practitioners 16: 127–134

Prescription Pricing Authority 1995 Annual report 1994–95. Prescription Pricing Authority, Newcastle

Record M C, Spencer J A, Jones R H, Jones K P 1994 General practitioners' views about the statutory annual practice report. British Medical Journal 309: 849–852

Royal College of General Practitioners. Office of Population Censuses and Surveys and Department of Health 1995 Morbidity statistics from general practice. Fourth national study 1991–1992. HMSO, London

Ryder B 1995 Screening for diabetic retinopathy. British Medical Journal 311: 207–208

Scobie S, Basnett I, McCartney P 1995 Can general practice data be used for needs assessment and health care planning in an inner London District? Journal of Public Health Medicine 17 (4) 475–483

Shanks J, Kheraj S, Fish S 1995 Better ways of assessing health needs in primary care. British Medical Journal 310: 480–481

Sheldon M G, Rector A L, Barnes P A 1984 The accuracy of age–sex registers in general practice. Journal of the Royal College of General Practitioners 31: 410–419

Squires N F, Beeching N J, Schlecht B J M, Ruben S 1995 An estimate of the prevalence of drug misuse in Liverpool and a spatial analysis of known addiction. Journal of Public Health Medicine 17: 103–109

Tapsfield J 1995 Wycombe Primary Care Prevention Project. Wycombe

Wilson A E, Pollock C, Weekes T, Dowell A 1995 Can general practice provide useful information? Evaluation of a primary health care project in northern England. Journal of Epidemiology and Community Health 49: 227–230

5

Assessing the needs of hard-to-reach groups

Mark Gabbay   John Gabbay

INTRODUCTION

Primary care teams are increasingly able to use needs assessment as a means of developing well-focused care programmes for major groups within their practices. (Gillam 1992, Shanks et al 1995). There is, however, a danger that this process will omit groups for whom the primary care team often finds it difficult to provide appropriate care. This chapter presents some points to consider as well as some practical guidelines and sources of information for primary health care teams and commissioners contemplating needs assessment in hard-to-reach groups. The most useful of these sources are discussed in the annotated bibliography.

WHAT ARE HARD-TO-REACH GROUPS?

There will inevitably be groups of people who require health care but are unlikely to come to their general practitioner (GP) to ask for it. They are also unlikely to come for health checks or screening. This may be for a number of possible reasons:

- They may misunderstand the nature and purpose of the services on offer, or may simply not understand the language that health professionals use. Such a communication barrier may not be simply due to their speaking a different language; it may be that the primary care team has failed to communicate effectively.

But the problems may be deeper:
- The group may not share the professionals' views about the importance of health care, or may feel alienated by the establishment whom they perceive GPs as representing.
- They may find the services on offer to be inappropriate or even threatening to themselves or their cultural standards.

The care offered may thus be physically, socially or culturally inaccessible or even frightening.

Such groups may include ethnic and cultural minorities, Travellers, refugees, and more or less defined subcultures of gay men, bisexuals and lesbians, substance abusers, sex workers, the homeless, or even adolescents.*

Debate as to whether such groups constitute separate homogeneous categories within the population or are merely 'outliers' of other groups would reveal much about one's attitudes to health care and society. Fortunately that debate is not relevant to the practical intentions of this chapter. We set out here merely to provide some pointers to good practice.

The principles by which the primary care team might overcome the barriers may also prove helpful in overcoming the fear of procedures such as cervical smears or injections which, though important, are not particular to minority groups. Thus, not only may specific needs assessment help to provide hard-to-reach groups* with better care, but the lessons learnt from that process can help to improve the care of more routine patients.

WHAT MAKES PRIMARY CARE INACCESSIBLE TO SUCH GROUPS?
Reasons for not registering

The population concerned may not have registered with any practice, which may wish to get them to do so. The desire to improve their health need not be the only motivation. There are likely to be other knock-on gains, for example the provision of medical care to a group of local drug misusers might lower crime and social stress in the neighbourhood, benefiting the health of other patients as a consequence. There will also be financial gains to the practice from increasing the list, which will help defray the extra costs involved. The practice may want to expand its list in competition with other local services or to enhance its image, matching its strengths to the needs of the local population. The practice may believe that it cannot reach its targets unless it manages to increase the uptake of preventative health measures amongst new groups of patients.

To encourage minority groups to register, it is important to consider their reasons for not having done so:

● Some people fear that registration will get them into trouble; for example, illegal immigrants worry that details may be passed on to the Home Office, while

substance abusers and sex workers fear criminal proceedings or that their children will be taken into care. Sometimes this is a legitimate fear – for example, GPs *are* a point of entry into the child protection process. But more often the fear is unfounded, and the practice will need to find a means of providing reassurance.
● They may have tried to register but been put off, for example by the attitudes of members of the team or patients in the waiting room.
● They may fear that the medical team will criticize them or try to get them to change their behaviour.
● They may not have got round to registering because they do not think they will need a doctor, or do not see it as a priority (e.g. students or people working away from home long term).
● They may simply not understand the UK health care system. This could be because they are used to a different health care system overseas, and nobody has explained the UK one to them.
● They may have assumed that somebody else would register them (e.g. students in a hall of residence).
● They may not understand how to register due to mental illness, learning difficulties or even just language difficulties.

Reasons for failing to take up services

Getting patients to register is only the first step. There may be a number of reasons for registered patients not using the services on offer:

● *Language difficulties.* There may not be any clinical member of staff with whom the patient can easily communicate. Interpreters may not be available, or may charge for the service (an increasing problem for one community group within the practice population of one of the authors). The available interpreter may induce embarrassment or shame or may be dominant, influencing what is said (e.g. a child, friend or stranger may put a woman off discussing sexual or gynaecological problems).
● *Patients may not know what is on offer because their language or literacy difficulties prevent them from doing so.* They may also have strong preconceptions that get in the way of them hearing what is said. Their view of what health care is, or of the role of the doctor, may be so far from what is being done that they cannot situate it within their sphere of reference (e.g. if they see the doctor as an authoritarian or a critical parent, then they will not interpret an inquiry about lifestyle in the intended way).
● *The patients' priorities are different.* They may not share health workers' views of the merits of prevention, health promotion, organized care of chronic disease, or continuity of care.

---

* Patients with mental illness and handicap are not considered as hard-to-reach groups within the definition of this chapter. Routine needs assessment and specialized services should be addressing them as individuals and perhaps as groups; however, their homelessness, ethnicity, sexuality, drug misuse, etc, may include them in one of the above categories. The annotated bibliography contains a section on mental illness and handicap which serves as an introduction to needs assessment issues with these groups.

- *Patients may find the service culturally insensitive.* This may sometimes be easily rectified by adapting the service (e.g. by using halal food in the meals on wheels, or by avoiding young women going to the houses of elderly Asian males), or it may be inevitable (e.g. believing that cocaine is harmless, or that smoking is so 'cool', that the consequences of later disease do not matter).

- *There may be a 'medical fear'.* Sometimes this problem is specific to the minority group; for example, Afro-Caribbean males may fear being labelled as schizophrenic if they present with psychological problems. But more usually it is a problem which is common to all medical groups but may need to be handled differently. For example, an awareness of the views and fears of intimate physical examination is essential for a successful targeting of cervical smear campaigns or for effective antenatal care within different cultural groups. This can be compounded, for example, by ignorance of the extent of, and views about, genital mutilation, which may be almost universal in adult women within certain ethnic minority groups.

HOW WILL NEEDS ASSESSMENT HELP?

Providers and purchasers of health care often find themselves 'limited to ... unaided judgment of which services would most benefit the health of local people' (Shanks et al 1995). It is easy to make false assumptions. In this section we briefly present some myths which health professionals commonly hold about hard-to-reach groups, and give examples of how information from local research or needs assessments has challenged those mistaken assumptions and led to improvements to the service.

Challenging assumptions through needs assessment

- *'Asians look after their own elderly'.* A project in Rochdale which investigated the needs of 'Asian elders' made use of a care manager in the local general practice who spoke the predominant Asian language and was a member of the community. It soon became clear that once access to available social services was eased in this way, and the elders and their carers felt more able to discuss their needs, carers began to request support services. This was supplemented by qualitative research with the target population highlighting cultural sensitivities and difficulties of access. Once the services were adapted to take account of this, the requests for such support soon began to match that of the local white population (Gupta & Greenbank 1993). Similar conclusions were reached in a large comprehensive study of minority ethnic elders' needs by Austin & Hartley (1993).

- *'Asians get unusual diseases'.* This may be so, but does not constitute the bulk of their health care needs. In southern Derbyshire, whilst 30% of all cases of tuberculosis were from ethnic minorities, there were only approximately 60 cases in total (Kenny et al 1994). Not only does that represent a tiny proportion of the morbidity in that group, but to concentrate on such diseases would not match the health concerns of the minority groups concerned. A radio phone-in during the London ethnic health project highlighted that the main concerns identified by Asians, namely skin disease, mental health, diabetes, asthma and infertility, did not match concurrent health education campaigns on tuberculosis, low-birth-weight babies and rickets targeted at the same group. Indeed, their main problem seemed to be accessing the care which the health authorities had assumed to be equally available to all (Hawthorne 1994). Over recent years there has been a tendency to concentrate on targeting services at unusual diseases in ethnic groups, e.g. high-profile initiatives to deal with thalassaemia amongst Afro-Caribbeans. Whilst this may be important, the health service should not neglect to concentrate resources where they will be most effective, targeting diabetes, hypertension and stroke prevention, which will affect a much higher proportion of the Afro-Caribbean population.

- *'Drug users do not want health care, and all their ills are drug related'.* General practice-based research has countered this view (Robertson 1985, Gabbay 1995). A questionnaire survey focusing on contact with GPs by opiate misusers attending a community drug team revealed a widespread desire amongst the misusers for access to primary health care services in addition to care focused on their drug problem (Gabbay et al 1996). An audit carried out in the practice of one of the authors (MG) showed that the GPs' preoccupation with the prescription of methadone and misuse behaviour resulted in low levels of immunization, cervical smears and health checks. Recognition of this fact catalysed a multidisciplinary drug misuse clinic, with a protocol including preventive healthcare. It is hoped that this will also enable 'routine' primary care to be separated from matters related to methadone prescription. Research is under way which should show if this is successful.

- *'Ethnic minority groups with particular health care needs related to their origin are "black"'.* Research into the standardized mortality ratios of Irish first- and second-generation immigrants shows them to be higher than controls, and that this is so does not seem to be satisfactorily accounted for by socioeconomic factors or genetic pre-disposition (Raftery et al 1990, Harding & Balarajan 1996). During the surveying of ethnic minority elders in South Glamorgan, it became clear that 'white' groups (Arabic speaking, Greek and Eastern European) had specific and different needs which were also not being met. Thus, it is clear that the provision of services to target health needs for ethnic minorities may require thinking beyond assumptions about skin colour.

● *'Adolescents will not want to discuss contraception'*. A survey of young people's health projects interviewed users (Allen 1991) who were indeed very keen to discuss these issues, but felt unable to do so within general practice settings because of their fears about lack of confidentiality. Similar concerns have been show in other studies (Ladipo 1994, McElnay & Cruikshank 1994).

● *'Our patch has no ethnic minority health care problems'*. Routine information can often be misleading. For example, ethnic group statistics derived from the census identified Gateshead as having the lowest proportion of ethnic minorities in the UK. However, orthodox Jews were not counted as an ethnic minority in the census but have clearly defined health care needs related to their culture (Fallon & Jones 1996). In fact, Gateshead has the largest strictly orthodox Jewish community in the UK. A health needs assessment study of this group discovered high birth rates, but low uptake of well woman screening and child immunization, the latter two in contrast with previous UK studies of Jews' health needs, perhaps reflecting the relative economic deprivation within the Gateshead community.

● *'Gay men with HIV and their carers are well informed about AIDS and the services available'*. This is not always so, and Bissell (1994) found that people with HIV were unsure how to access services.

These examples show that local research can provide information that runs counter to the assumptions of health care professionals, and informs the quality of their decision making both as providers and commissioners/purchasers. Such work may highlight the need for enhanced accessibility, for example by:

● Meeting language needs, e.g. interpreters, leaflet and invitation letter translation
● Training staff in cultural sensitivity
● Providing specific services including outreach clinics.

Such knowledge may also help primary care teams to formulate appropriate service specifications for the providers of secondary care to patients who have specific cultural needs.

WHY IS A DIFFERENT APPROACH TO NEEDS ASSESSMENT REQUIRED?

The techniques for needs assessment described elsewhere in this book may not yield useful results for the groups we are considering in this chapter. Routine information usually fails to identify, or even include, them. General surveys will almost certainly fail to reach some

of these groups, or will fail to elicit responses. Unless correctly handled, focus groups or other means of gathering local opinions will not adequately involve some of the hard-to-reach groups. The strengths and weaknesses of various techniques applied in a small community needs assessment have recently been discussed (Murray & Graham 1995).

GETTING STARTED
Defining the group

The first step is to decide which group(s) one has even begun to focus on and why. Minority groups are heterogeneous. They are also difficult to define, and one's definition will rarely match the way they perceive themselves. It is important not to select a group which does not recognize itself as such. Bangladeshis and Sikhs would not necessarily take kindly to being lumped together as 'Asians'. To do so may be to alienate them before beginning. There have been strong critiques of the trend to categorize groups on ethnic grounds (Bhopal et al 1991, Sheldon & Parker 1992, Benzeval et al 1995, Bhopal 1995). Often the groups studied are poorly defined and may be more varied within the grouping on many social, cultural, economic and health measures than they are divergent from the White population with which they are being compared. Some of the reports cited in the annotated bibliography refer to 'Black and minority ethnic groups' as this was the aim of the project concerned; thus their findings may need to be applied with caution amongst your target population, but the task of checking out their applicability can be fairly straightforward.

Building on the work of others

It is important to do some early background reading. There is no point reinventing the wheel. Start with what may already have been done elsewhere and then consider how the findings may apply to the population and the services offered. The annotated bibliography gives examples of recent health needs assessments amongst minority groups. The findings and recommendations as well as the methodological approaches provide a starting point to initial planning and discussion as one begins to think about current service provision and feasible changes. The bibliography may also highlight useful literature sources of a more general nature. For a wider search, use the librarian at the local medical or university library, or consult *Medline*. The King's Fund 'Share project' publishes material on ethnic minority needs assessment. This includes a newsletter, guides to literature including reports, and lists of professionals involved in such work in the UK, obtainable free of charge. The local community health council may be a valuable resource, and keen to help. Ask local purchasers and/or providers (1) what they are doing or have done, and (2) what they know of work being done elsewhere.

Considering the potential impact

An early discussion within the practice team will be very useful. Discussions may reveal more prejudice in the practice than was acknowledged. Consider how the bulk of patients may react, how much that matters to the team, and how any potential changes resulting from the needs assessment may impact on the current priorities for the practice. It may be too disruptive of 'ordinary' services to adapt to a particular group's needs. The team should also consider possible ethical dilemmas, e.g. is it ethical to ask drug users to find others, even when it is known they are involved in illegal activities? However, involvement in such work can be therapeutic, as was shown in one group of misusers involved in peer education and needs assessment who stiffened in their resolve to come off drugs (Bottomley et al 1995). One may be considered to be supporting illegal behaviour (e.g. illegal immigration, drug use or under-age sex), or to be undermining other public service authorities (e.g. social services who may wish to take a drug user's children into care).

Agreeing the scale of the task

Do not try and do too much. Start small and simple, looking for change that is possible. Early discussions with primary care providers, health authority managers and public health specialists should ensure that realistic goals are set. Most practices have the resources to carry out a fairly simple exploration of the needs of hard-to-reach groups. It is worth remembering, however, that to carry out a full health needs assessment into minority groups even in a local area may be very expensive. Few if any practices would have access to the necessary resources; for example, to conduct a good qualitative survey of an ethnic group for example would require a researcher costing over £20 000 (Hughes et al 1995). Moreover, it would need to be determined that it would be cost-effective for the practice to implement potential changes from within existing resources, or whether the changes are likely to attract personnel and financial support from elsewhere. But this sort of work is an ideal area for joint development initiatives between primary care and others, for example the local health authority, the regional research and development directorate, academic departments of primary care or public health or appropriate charities. The results may be applicable elsewhere, adding to the quality of care on a wider scale. For all these reasons, and even for a small project, it might be helpful to discuss it early on with the local public health team, or academic department of general practice or public health, rather than setting out on the task alone.

It is quite probable that the early stages of readings and discussions may have answered questions, and that such information, perhaps along with an estimate of the size of the local target population, will enable enhancement of the service sufficiently for a better dialogue to develop with the target group, and hence proceed to meet the objective of improving the service they receive. However, one may wish to carry out some local information gathering, either of statistical data, or of qualitative data. The following practical guide contains information applicable to such simple local needs assessment projects.

CONDUCTING A LOCAL STUDY

Data from work done elsewhere may well apply to the target population, and it may be much more feasible to check the extent to which they are relevant, by conducting a brief survey of health professionals and others as outlined in the next section, than to gather new data. If other people's data is used, it is important to have sufficient information on how the data was gathered to be able to form a judgement of their reliability, validity and applicability. The pros and cons of different methods are outlined in this chapter and elsewhere in this book.

Discussions with providers, purchasers and consumers

It will be useful to ask colleagues in a systematic way about their knowledge of the group in question, the services currently provided, and the scope for improvements. Many assessments of needs in primary care have only involved collecting the views of service providers and purchasers. This has its biases, but is relatively cheap, and may reveal a wealth of useful knowledge and data. Furthermore, such a process is likely to enhance the enthusiasm of these same people when it comes to making changes.

Consulting with the wider primary health care team may be very informative. Health visitors and midwives in one's own team, for example, may know more about a target population. Practice staff usually live in the community, and have considerable knowledge and experience of the area and its people. Simply employing people in the practice who belong to the ethnic group one wishes to contact may greatly increase their view of its accessibility, and provide interpreters who are part of the team. Colleagues in other primary care teams may also provide information. Talk to purchasers and providers, especially services who may have experience with the group, e.g. the local community or regional drug team. It might also be helpful to consult the local authority social services, housing, or education (e.g. school nursing service) departments.

Patients or other members of the group who are already known to the practice are a useful starting point. Patients can also be contacted by advertising in the surgery or by personal contact, telephone or letter. Talk to the Community Health Council and to relevant voluntary organizations, community leaders and groups, pressure groups, outreach workers, hostels, etc. They may have an interest in the subject, collect useful data, and have potential expertise and volunteers.

It may be that there is still not enough information to meet the objectives. Perhaps the population's circumstances are different or unknown, or the knowledge base about comparable groups poor. In that case, a fuller needs assessment may be needed, for which the following guide may be helpful.

Routine data sources

If more needs to be known about the size of the population in question, there are several potential data sources. Their statistical drawbacks, and relevance to the local area, need to be considered. Box 5.1 is a guide to these sources and their limitations. Other methods of gathering specific data prospectively are dealt with in the next section.

Collecting local data

McKeganey (1995) has recently challenged the attitudes about the relative worth of quantitative versus qualitative data. Well-conducted small qualitative surveys can be excellent for gaining insights into service provision and use, though not necessarily generalizable, especially if used in isolation. There may be scope for a larger, quantitative survey – for example to determine the prevalence of a group in a local area. However, the findings may not be generalizable unless the right steps are taken to ensure the sample selection is random, and includes sufficient numbers of relevant subgroups.

If a survey is to be conducted, all the caveats about keeping needs assessment simple and within resource limits apply. Get expert help early. Explore the possibilities of jointly resourcing such work with others, as good surveys can be difficult and expensive, but if well designed can be extremely helpful.

Box 5.1   Routine data sources

Local public health department
These are useful guides through this potential maze of statistics, and will have regional and local datasets including:

- Mortality (including standardized mortality ratios)
- Morbidity statistics (particularly in respect of health of the nation targets).

The annual public health reports may be a good starting place.

Providers' data on activity and service utilization
May include ethnic monitoring figures.

Census data
Provide information down to enumeration district level (Majeed et al 1995) that includes:

- Age and gender demographics
- Ethnic origin of the head of households
- Basic socioeconomic measures.

Potential problems include:

Differences between the target population and the wider local population
- Certain groups under-represented during the census data collection
- The ecological fallacy, i.e. that the characteristics of places and areas do not necessarily represent the characteristics of an individual who lives there (Scrivener & Lloyd 1995).

Practice-held data
That is, information routinely collected in patient notes on:

- Morbidity (e.g. mental health register)*
- Demographic data
- Ethnic and social characteristics of the target population.

Unfortunately, data are often insufficient to meet practices' requirements for this purpose, but some prospective data collection at least for newly registering patients may help, e.g. language(s) in which the patient is able to communicate comfortably (spoken and/or written).

* As suggested by Kendrick et al (1994). This is being developed in the practice of one of the authors (MG) to highlight patients with severe and relapsing mental illness. This enables a needs assessment of patients identified in this way as well as a recall and monitoring system. The local mental health services should be developing needs assessment as part of their care programme approach, which can be adapted for primary care use.

Getting further access

Work with a friendly contact, perhaps a patient, who can give some insight into the target group's culture. Initial contacts may be used to make further contact with the group. If a patient is used in this way, consider how this may affect the therapeutic relationship, e.g. if one discusses these issues with a drug misuser for whom one prescribes, this influences future consultation processes.

Try and find out who some of the opinion leaders are, and those with influence in the community without whose support it may be difficult to gain access into the group. Consider the need to balance this potential sample with contacts amongst others within the community who differ from their 'community leaders', for example, religious observance, gender or economic status. There are potential biases in most methods. An extensive study of qualitative research with 'Asian' communities has explored these dilemmas in some detail (Rai 1995). It is important to consider the possible limitations, including the representativeness of informants and how the power balance may have prevented honest and open communication. This strategy also risks potential adverse effects on the people that are asked, alienating them from their peer group or close contacts, which may increase their own stress – being seen as collaborators with what their peers regard as the enemy.

Snowballing

This is a useful technique for enlarging the sample. Use informants to provide the names of others who may then be approached and interviewed and also asked for contacts, building up a sample among hard-to-reach groups. The sample may be biased but can be improved by randomly selecting those for follow-up from suggested names. This technique in a study of ethnic minority elders opened up new areas of concern in groups not thought to have a problem, who were then accessed and interviewed (Austin & Hartley 1993). The snowball technique has been used very effectively in the field of drug misuse, using current drug users as 'privileged access interviewers' (Griffiths et al 1993, Power 1994, Bottomley et al 1995). It can be particularly useful with very hard-to-reach groups such as sex workers (McKeganey et al 1994).

Specific registers

It may be worth constructing lists of people in the target group. The practice list may be searched for names associated with specific ethnic groups. Retrospective lists of ethnic minority surnames may work well for patients originating in the Indian subcontinent (Ecob & Williams 1991) and Chinese and Vietnamese populations, but is more problematic for Africans where even within the same family group surnames may differ (Local Government Management Board 1995) and impractical for Afro-Caribbeans whose surnames are not sufficiently distinguishable from those of other groups (Hughes et al 1995). Think laterally and consult 'informants' for ideas. In Gateshead the researchers consulted with community leaders, who suggested the Kosher milkman's list as a source of names and addresses of the previously unidentified large group of orthodox Jews which could then be searched on the practice computer for health data (Fallon & Jones 1996). In Hull the research team used the *Yellow Pages* to select randomly 30 Chinese takeaways, and matched them with 30 English fish and chip shops in order to compare the employees' use of, and views

about, health care (Watt et al 1993). A combination of methods including geographical spotting, i.e. targeting streets with large numbers of the relevant population, lists from affiliations to religious, social or pressure groups (to correct for potential biases) and snowballing may all be required to produce a list. Registers of substance abusers in contact with the practice may be compiled from a practice audit of methadone prescribing, or figures from regional or national drug addict databases. Lists of Travellers who have been in contact with the practice can be compiled. Community organizations, hostels, outreach workers, posters or leaflets in places frequented by members of the target group, e.g. youth clubs for teenagers or needle exchanges/pharmacies for drug misusers, may all potentially be sources of contacts within the target population. Lam & Green (1994) obtained their contact list from addresses known to the local Vietnamese refugee project from which they randomly selected their sample.

There are ethical dilemmas in constructing such lists and patients may resent it, so it is necessary to check. Secret police, after all, keep such lists too. Compiling lists from other than practice-held data should therefore involve negotiation with community groups and representatives if only to allay fears. Despite their practical and ethical problems, such lists may make audit and research far easier. Using DHA or registration lists can be disheartening as they are often inaccurate and out of date to a degree that results in unacceptably high levels of wrong addresses (Hughes et al 1995, E Elliot, personal communication), though computerized links may improve this. Furthermore, in hard-to-reach groups many of the target population may not be registered. Using the electoral register may miss out those in the group most at risk and difficult to access, as they are unlikely to have registered to vote. The Salford PHRRC project (Elliott & Bennett 1996) initially carried out a mini census in streets which they had identified as rich in the target population. This resulted in a very high response rate to the qualitative survey, as contact had already been made during the census, and the interviewers were not 'cold calling'.

Collecting the information

Semi-structured interviews with randomly selected populations with statistical corrections for bias probably represent the gold standard, but studies suggest that minority group members, if able to write their name and read relatively small print, are able to give satisfactory health needs assessment information via a written questionnaire (Sullivan et al 1995). Ramirez and colleagues (1996) conducted their survey of the health care needs of lesbians, gay men and bisexuals by handing out their questionnaire at major events for that community. Whilst recognizing that the sample would be largely biased to those who were 'out', they could also target minority subgroups such as women, the Black community and disabled people easily, to enrich their information.

If a survey is conducted, one should consider carefully whom to employ as fieldworker, and in particular the balance between their research skills and their knowledge of and credibility with the group being investigated. It is also necessary to ensure that they have the appropriate training, support and supervision. Beware of them using their position in an exploitative way, or being seen as potentially doing so by the people they contact. It is important not to dabble in unknown territory, which can lead to difficulties for the practice. However, if preliminary background work is done as above it is likely that support and advice from others with sufficient relevant experience will help to avoid such pitfalls. Many of the reports and papers listed in the annotated bibliography include sections on the recruitment and support of fieldworkers (e.g. Shah et al 1993, Griffiths et al 1993, Power 1994, Rai 1995).

Observation – participant and non-participant

Data gathering need not be a complicated business. A lot can be learnt from simply taking the time to observe systematically and objectively what happens in practice when the team interacts (or fails to interact) with the hard-to-reach groups. Such observation can be conducted within the day-to-day practice (participant observation), but this technique runs the risk of being subjective and selective. To avoid selection and recall bias, therefore, one should be rigorous and systematic in deciding what data to collect, and record the data fully and faithfully and preferably as soon as they have been observed (Hammersley & Atkinson 1983). If several of the team do the same it will not only help to reduce subjectivity, but provide a fruitful basis for agreeing the practical implications of results which have been observed.

Alternatively, spend time observing each others' interactions (non-participant observation), or even arrange with colleagues elsewhere to do an exchange visit to observe other practices. Perhaps a local member of the hard-to-reach group, or the community health council, or – say – the local drug misuse team, could be invited to observe how things are done. Audit within the practice might also provide a useful vehicle for improving how the needs of the minority groups are met.

Interviews will require an interviewer able to speak the language of the target group, which can have unexpected advantages and disadvantages. The Hull research into Chinese and white catering workers, unfortunately,

coincided with VAT inspector enquiries, and community suspicions were only allayed by the team's Chinese researcher. Conversely, some people feel ashamed when discussing health issues with a member of their own community, fearing judgement and a lack of confidentiality (Rai 1995, E Elliott, personal communication). It may be very important to have an interviewer of the same gender (Hughes et al 1995, Rai 1995). The interview situation and appearance of the interviewer will significantly affect the response of the interviewee (Davies 1992, Rai 1995). It may be possible to access trained interviewers (Rai 1995).

Questionnaires may be used, but all the caveats about survey design (see Chs 2 and 8) apply equally to qualitative as to quantitative surveys, and again it is advisable to get help from a relevant local academic department, or from the Office of Population Censuses and Surveys (OPCS)*. Many projects described in the sources referenced in this chapter have already translated questionnaires and information into a variety of languages, which may help in the desired study.

Focus groups are commonly used as a formal technique for obtaining views (see Ch. 8). In constructing such a group, it is necessary to be especially careful about balancing the involvement of local community leaders with the views of their 'opponents', or those alienated from them (see above under the heading 'Defining the group'). Some local authorities, for example Salford, already have established neighbourhood discussion groups. It may be worthwhile dividing the group up by age and gender, to free up the discussion (Williams 1993). The group will need at least two facilitators fluent in the relevant languages, one to facilitate, one to take notes, although making notes in English is not thought to affect the data quality adversely and simplifies subsequent analysis (Hughes et al 1995). The areas for discussion may be obvious. It is useful to have some idea of the areas to be explored, and a working knowledge of other similar studies elsewhere is extremely helpful, while retaining an open mind. It is a good idea to tape the groups, if they agree to it.

Postal or geographic surveys can be used, but are unlikely to be feasible in primary care, unless supported by larger organizations such as health authorities. It is more likely that outreach-type work may be necessary, perhaps using members of the target community as co-workers to enhance acceptability (Bottomley et al 1995, Fay et al 1995).

Rapid appraisal is a flexible approach, adaptable to the data collection required for looking at minority groups. It entails obtaining interviews on the needs of the com-

---

* The Health Survey Advice Centre, OPCS Social Survey Division, St Catherine's House, London WC2B 6JP.

munity from key informants, secondary data collection from various sources, observation and mapping, both social and geographical, confirming data obtained through triangulation (Ong et al 1991, Murray et al 1995, Ong 1994). This may be a relatively quick and practical method of carrying out a more detailed needs assessment. It is more likely to be successful where the target group is largely confined to a particular area rather than scattered and fairly invisible.

CONCLUSION

Needs assessment amongst minority groups in primary care can be relatively straightforward (e.g. Pistrang 1990, Hadjicharitou et al 1994, Williams 1993, Tang & Cuninghame 1994), successfully enabling change and inspiring the professionals involved. It is, however,

essential to feed back the findings and planned service changes derived from the needs assessment process to the members of the community in question. The literature is full of reports of disillusioned minority groups complaining about answering yet another set of questions when nothing ever changes. Insensitive though well-intentioned interventions can be counter-productive (Webb 1995).

Box 5.2 presents an outline of a 'simple' study as an example of what can be done easily and cheaply. The lessons potentially gained from such work have relevance across the whole spectrum of health care provision and purchasing. The results can be rewarding not only for the target group, but also for the practice as a whole. By enhancing the health of those in greatest need, standards of health care are likely to be enhanced across the board.

Box 5.2 Outline of 'simple' project. (Based on Hadjicharitou et al (1994).)

1. Planning
Practice and public health physician meet to discuss possible subjects for investigation, the questions they wish to answer and the methods for meeting the agreed objectives. They decide on a service needs assessment of 'Asian' patients.

2. Workload indicators for study chosen in this case
- Consultations
- Prescription items
- Booked appointments versus 'extras'
- Home visits, including night visits.

3. Method
Asian name list drawn up, checked against the DHA- and census data-derived estimate of numbers. One in five sample of notes studied with age–sex comparison of non-Asian patients. Consultation rates, prescription data, appointment and visit data checked.

4. Pragmatic *Medline* literature search and review
Of research on effects of ethnicity on consultation rates and service usage.

5. Initial contact with community health council link-worker
Background information and snowballing of other contacts. Five non-patients interviewed about Asian populations service needs

and background information about the community profile. Patient interviews. Three patients interviewed (open technique) about:
- Length of and reasons for registration with the practice
- Preferred GP (if any)
- Characteristics of good and bad GPs
- What is good about the service for Asian patients and what improvements could be made.

6 Meeting
With all three GPs, the practice manager, the public health physician, and two of the three interviewed patients. Initial community contact (community health council link-worker) unable to attend. Findings discussed including unmet needs.

7. Changes
GPs meet in the following week, and draw up an action plan covering:
- Further research requirements
- Training needs
- Translation of leaflets by local schoolchildren
- Proposal to investigate the recruitment of a fluent Punjabi-speaking member of the staff as a pilot project with the health commission
- Setting up of regular patient participation meetings.

ANNOTATED BIBLIOGRAPHY

The following list contains useful literature and contacts which may provide a guide to some of the more useful sources available.

Ethnic minorities

Austin R, Hartley B 1993 Towards a good old age? The GOAL project. Racial Equality Council, Glamorgan, UK. *Comprehensive report of a large survey of the health needs of people of ethnic minority over the age of 50 years. Includes a discussion of the methodology, useful details about running the project, and its findings.*

Balarajan R 1995 Ethnicity and variations in the nation's health. Health Trends 27: 114–119. *This paper examines the relationship between ethnicity and mortality indicators in the health of the nation white paper.*

Camden and Islington Health Authority 1993 Health needs assessment of black and minority ethnic people in Camden and Islington, London, UK. Camden and Islington Health Authority, London. *Substantial and richly referenced review with conclusions and recommendations for commissioners.*

Gill P, Scrivener G, Lloyd D, Dowell T, 1995 The effect of patient ethnicity on prescribing rates. Health Trends 27: 111–114. *Large survey, based on data from the General Household Survey.*

Hadjicharitou C, Tabner J A, Smith D A, Ayres P J 1994 Towards a better service with our Asian patients. Public Health in Primary Care Report 2. Wakefield Healthcare, Wakefield, UK. *A joint GP/public health project on needs amongst 'Asian' patients in a practice that reviews workload and user views; relatively simple and practical methodology.*

Hughes A O, Fenton S, Hine C E 1995 Strategies for sampling black and ethnic minority populations. Journal of Public Health Medicine 17(2): 187–192. *A description of project design and sampling methods.*

Karmi G, McKeigue P 1993 The ethnic health bibliography. NE and NW Thames Regional Health Authority, London. *Comprehensive bibliography up to and including (in part) 1993.*

Kenny C, Qurban A, Cassidy M 1994 A review of the health needs of people from black and minority ethnic groups in southern Derbyshire. Derbyshire FHSA, Derby. *Approaches the issue from reviewing progress with previous recommendations and specific projects to address the needs of ethnic minorities, and thus may stimulate ideas for potential projects.*

Lam T, Green J 1994 Primary health care and the Vietnamese community: a survey in Greenwich. Health and Social Care in the Community 2: 293–299. *Interview based, highlighting language, mental health problems, and ophthalmic service needs.*

Li P-L 1992 Health needs of the Chinese population. In: Ahmad W I U (ed) The politics of 'race' and health. Race Relations Research Unit, Bradford and Ilkely Community College, Bradford. *Historical and literature review of the UK Chinese community, and report of an initiative to meet their needs.*

Nguyen-Van-Tam J, Simpson J, Madeley R, Davies L 1995 Health care experiences of Vietnamese families in Nottingham. Health Trends 27: 106–110. *Presents findings of a large interview survey amongst Vietnamese refugees about their use of and experiences with primary health care services.*

Pistrang N 1990 Leaping the culture gap. Health Service Journal 100: 878–879. *Interviews of providers of services within the London Chinese community, looking at mental health needs.*

Rai D K 1995 In the margins, current practices in qualitative social research with Asian communities. Papers in Social Research 2. University of Humberside, Hull. *Comprehensive study of current practices in qualitative research methods with Asian communities, rich in data and guidelines.*

Shah L, Harvey I, Coyle E 1993 The health and social care needs of ethnic minorities in South Glamorgan. Report of Centre for Applied Public Health Medicine. University of Wales College of Medicine, Cardiff. *Contains a useful discussion of methodology and useful data.*

Share 1994 Needs assessment: bibliography. King's Fund Centre, London.

Share 1994 Needs assessment: list of contacts. King's Fund Centre, London. *The Share project at the King's Fund provides extensive lists of projects, contacts and publications. Using these it is possible to obtain personal contacts and written information which will save reinventing the wheel, and provide guidance and support.*

Tang M, Cuninghame C 1994 Ways of saying. Health Service Journal 104: 28–30. *Preliminary report of focus group discussions on the needs of Vietnamese women and elders.*

Watt I S, Howel D, Lo L 1993 The health care experience and health behaviour of the Chinese: a survey based in Hull. Journal of Public Health Medicine 15(2): 129–136. *Comparison between Chinese and 'White' catering workers of experience, use, and views about primary health care.*

Wigham L 1993 Access to primary health care services by the Somalian population of South Glamorgan. South Glamorgan FHSA, Cardiff. *Morbidity data, background to and results of health initiatives with Somalian population.*

Williams G 1993 The health and social needs of the Yemeni community in Eccles and Salford. Salford and Trafford Health Authority, Salford. *Methodology and results of focus group discussions with Yemeni people.*

Adolescents

Allen I 1991 Family planning and pregnancy counselling projects for young people. Policy Studies Institute, London. *This book reports the findings of a study of three health projects aimed at young adults and teenagers. It is comprehensive and rich in quotes of staff and users.*

Denyer S 1994 Sexual health, annual report of the director of public health. Wirral Health, Tranmere. *A report of teenagers' sexual health needs.*

Jacobson L D, Wilkinson C E 1994 Review of teenage health: time for a new direction. British Journal of General Practice 44: 420–424. *Comprehensive literature review including research findings and reports of interventions.*

Kai R, Speed M, Ryan H 1992 (a) Today's young adults. (b) Tomorrow's young adults. Health Education Authority, London. *Large reports of a MORI survey of 9–15 and 16–19 year olds looking at attitudes and behaviour with respect to diet, alcohol, drugs, smoking, exercise and sexual behaviour. The data are also presented divided into regions.*

Ladipo N 1994 Assessment of health needs of teenagers in a GP practice. Bury and Rochdale Health Authority, Bury. *Practice-based survey of teenagers' health needs.*

McElnay C, Cruikshank R 1994 Contraceptive services in Manchester, a health needs assessment project. Manchester Health Authority, Manchester. *Report of teenagers' contraception needs.*

Substance abusers

Bottomley T, Smith M, Wibberley C 1995 Peer education amongst crack users, not so cracked. Druglink May/June: 9–12. *Although the project described was the development of peer education, the information available from this group is informative on the practicalities of privileged access interviews, and the leaflets devised from this work are of high quality.*

Griffiths P, Gossop M, Powis B, Strang J 1993 Researching hidden populations of drug users by privileged access interviewers: methodological and practical issues. Addiction 88: 1617–1626. *Discusses the practicalities of qualitative research amongst substance abusers in some detail.*

Power R 1994 Some methodological and practical implications of employing drug users as indigenous fieldworkers. In: Boulton M (ed) Challenge and innovation: methodological advances in social research on HIV/AIDS. Taylor and Francis, London. *See previous comment.*

Gay community/HIV

Bissell P 1994 Responding to the community care needs of people with HIV disease and their carers in Salford. Report of the Public Health Research and Resource Centre, Salford. *Presents findings and service recommendations from a district survey of people with HIV and their carers.*

London Lesbians in Health Care 1995 Lesbian health matters. The Wheel, London. *Training video and teaching pack primary care teams which aims to promote a more accessible and sympathetic service for this group.*

Ramirez A 1996 Assessing lesbian, gay and bisexual health care needs, draft preliminary report. Thames Valley University, Ealing, London. *Comprehensive report including a rich bibliography and methodology discussion.*

Homeless

Connelly J, Crown J (Eds) 1994 Homelessness and Ill Health. Royal College of Physicians, London. *Comprehensive report in book form on the health problems and needs of homeless people.*

Gaulton-Berks L 1994 Homeless choices. Nursing Times 90(34): 52–54. *Concerns the needs of homeless women, including focus group findings.*

Travellers

Fay R, Kevaney J, Charles A 1995 Report on the travellers' health project. Dublin Travellers' Education and Development Group, Dublin. *Describes the development of a primary care service including the use of traveller women as facilitators. Results of needs assessments presented.*

Hennink M, Cooper P, Diamond I 1995 Primary health care needs of travelling people in Wessex. Working paper 95–01. Department of Social Statistics, University of Southampton, Southampton. *Covers primary health care needs assessments of different types of traveller, including the sexual health needs of 'new age' travellers.*

Mental illness and learning disability/handicap

Audit Commission 1994 Finding a place, a review of mental health services for adults. HMSO, London. *Comprehensive review of adult mental health services.*

Ellahi R, Hatfield C 1992 Research into the needs of Asian families caring for someone with mental handicap. Mental Handicap 20: 134–136. *Presents results of questionnaire survey of mainly Pakistani origin families with a child with mental handicap, focusing on communication with professionals and their knowledge and experience of care facilities. It highlighted the need for a Punjabi speaker in the team as most carers would be unable to read a leaflet in Urdu.*

Goh S, Holland A J 1994 A framework for commissioning services for people with learning disabilities. Journal of Public Health Medicine 16(3): 279–285. *Outlines the application of the World Health Organization's model of disability as a framework for conceptualizing the needs of people with a learning disability.*

Nothard A 1993 Uptake of services for people with learning disabilities from Black and minority ethnic communities in Leeds. Leeds Community Mental Health Trust, Leeds. *Findings of a survey of service uptake by people with a learning disability and their carers from ethnic minorities. Includes the questionnaire used.*

REFERENCES

Benzeval M, Judge K, Smaje C 1995 Beyond class, race, ethnicity: deprivation and health in Britain. Health Services Research 30(1) (part 2): 151–177

Bhopal R S 1995 Unpublished manuscript of paper to Society for Social Medicine. Journal of Epidemiology and Community Health 49: 534–554

Bhopal R S, Phillimore P, Kohli H S 1991 Inappropriate use of the term 'Asian': an obstacle to ethnicity and health research. Journal of Public Health Medicine 13(4): 244–246

Davies J B 1992 The myth of addiction. Harwood Academic Press, Reading

Ecob R, Williams R 1991 Sampling Asian minorities to assess health and welfare. Journal of Epidemiology and Community Health 45: 93–101

Elliott E, Bennett S 1996 Linking information on needs and service options in NHS purchasing: a case study of mental health needs in two contrasting population health groups: interim report. Salford Public Health Research and Resources Centre, Salford

Fallon P V, Jones K P 1996 Assessing primary health care needs in an orthodox Jewish community in Gateshead: interim report. Department of Primary Healthcare, University of Newcastle, Newcastle

Gabbay M B 1995 Dealing with drug misuse. Journal of the Royal Society of Health 115(6): 391–394

Gabbay M B, Smith M, Dawkes M 1996 A study of drug misusers' contacts with general practitioners. Addiction Research 4(2): 125–137

Gillam S J 1992 Assessing the health care needs of populations – the general practitioners contribution. British Journal of General Practice 42: 404–405

Gupta P, Greenbank J 1993 Asian elders care management project report. Social Services Department, Rochdale

Hammersley M, Atkinson P 1983 Ethnography principles in practice. Routledge, London

Harding S, Balarajan R 1996 Patterns of mortality in second generation Irish living in England and Wales: longitudinal study. British Medical Journal 312: 1389–1392

Hawthorne K 1994 Accessibility and use of health care services in the British Asian community. Family Practice 11(4): 453–459

Kendrick T, Burns T, Freeling P, Sibbald B 1994 Provision of care to general practice patients with disabling long-term mental illness: a survey in 16 practices. British Journal of General Practice 44: 301–305

Local Government Management Board 1995 Learning from African Families. LGMB, Luton

McKeganey N 1995 Quantitative and qualitative research in the addictions: an unhelpful divide. Addiction 90: 749–751

McKeganey N, Barnard M, Bloor M 1994 How many prostitutes? Epidemiology out of ethnography. In: Boulton M (ed) Challenge and innovation: methodological advances in social research on HIV/AIDS. Taylor and Francis, London, pp. 111–122

Majeed F A, Cook D G, Poloniecki J, Martin D 1995 Using data from the 1991 census. British Medical Journal 310: 1511–1514

Murray S A, Graham L J C 1995 Practice based health needs assessment: use of four methods in a small neighbourhood. British Medical Journal 310: 1443–1448

Murray S A, Tapson J, Turnbull L, McCallum J, Little A 1994 Listening to local voices: adapting rapid appraisal to assess health and social needs in general practice. British Medical Journal 308: 698–700

Ong B N 1994 Prioritising needs with communities: rapid appraisal methodologies in health. In: Popay J, Williams G (eds) Researching the peoples health. Routledge, London, p 58

Ong B N, Humphries G, Annett H, Rifkin S 1991 Rapid appraisal in an urban setting, an example from the developed world. Social Science and Medicine 32: 900–915

Raftery J, Jones D R, Rosato M 1990 The mortality of first and second generation Irish immigrants in the U.K. Social Science and Medicine 31(5): 577–584

Robertson J R 1985 Drug users in contact with general practice. British Medical Journal 290: 34–35

Scrivener G, Lloyd D C E F 1995 Allocating census data to general practice populations: implications for study of prescribing variation at practice level. British Medical Journal 311: 163–165

Shanks J, Kheraj S, Fish S 1995 Better ways of assessing health needs in primary care. British Medical Journal 310: 480–481

Sheldon T A, Parker H 1992 Race and ethnicity in health research. Journal of Public Health Medicine 14(2): 104–110

Sullivan L M, Kimberley A, Dukes M et al 1995 A comparison of various methods of collecting self-reported health outcomes data among low-income and minority patients. Medical Care 33 (4)(Suppl): AS183-AS194

Webb E, 1995 Sexual mores: female genital mutilation – a worldwide problem. British Journal of Sexual Medicine 22(6): 6–8

6

Epidemiologically based needs assessment

Andrew Stevens   Mike Sadler

INTRODUCTION

Epidemiologically based needs assessment was designed as a 'gold standard' of needs assessment, but recognizing the approaches of comparative and corporate assessment (see Box 1.2). In combination they are potentially very powerful. The epidemiological approach is scientific, quantitative and very time-consuming.

The term 'epidemiologically based needs assessment' is something of a misnomer. Epidemiologically based needs assessment in practice concerns not just the *incidence and prevalence* of disease, but also the *effectiveness* of the interventions available to deal with the disease. In many, if not most, instances the effectiveness of interventions is the more important consideration. Epidemiologically based needs assessment also always requires an understanding of *current services*. The term 'epidemiologically based needs assessment' was, however, established by the *Health Care Needs Assessment* series (Stevens and Raftery 1994), in which 20 different disease groups covering perhaps 30% of health care activity (by cost) in the UK were reviewed: diabetes mellitus, renal disease, stroke (acute cerebrovascular disease), lower respiratory disease, coronary heart disease, colorectal cancer, cancer of the lung, total hip replacement, total knee replacement, cataract surgery, hernia repair, varicose vein treatments, prostatectomy for benign prostatic hyperplasia, mental illness, dementia, alcohol misuse, drug abuse, people with learning disabilities, community child health services and family planning, abortion and fertility services. The object of that exercise was based on trying to assist the District Health Authorities (of which in 1990 there were about 200) to assess the health care needs of their population to inform health care purchasing arising from the National Health Service (NHS) Review. In many respects, the information needs of general practitioners (GPs) as purchasers of health care are very similar. The essence of good practice in both purchasing and providing care is to consider whether or not what is being done for patients is effective and to consider all potential patients whether visible or not.

The differences between GPs as purchasers and district health authorities as purchasers include:

1. The fact that GPs are both purchasers of secondary and providers of primary health care (and the two are not necessarily always distinct)
2. The smaller population base with which GPs are concerned
3. The focus GPs often have with individual patients either as individuals, or as exemplars of particular health service problems
4. The different staff and support available to GPs as opposed to health commissions
5. The fact that at the primary care consultation, 'problems' are not necessarily translated or translatable into 'disease' groups
6. Recognition of the important role of primary care not just to treat people but also *both* to provide information and reassurance to the patient *and* to act as a filter to reserve secondary care for when it is really needed.

However, the central tenets of epidemiologically based needs assessment are to some extent even more applicable to primary care purchasing. Prime amongst these is that it is more efficient to get the best information from the literature, and to some extent also from routine data, collectively just once rather than replicating the exercise many times. The shortcut of needs assessment material produced for district health authorities to interpret locally, thus avoiding their having to seek it individually, applies even more to general practice.

Epidemiologically based needs assessment is a 'gold standard' on the basis that 'the need for health care' could be interpreted as the population's ability to benefit from health care. This is quite distinct from the 'need for health' which is more nebulous. From the point of view of purchasers of health care the ability to benefit is critical. Each component of this definition of the need for health care is important:

● The *population's* ability to benefit from health care equals the sum of individuals' ability to benefit. For many health problems this can be deduced from epidemiological studies, although smaller populations (i.e. patient groups) can be calculated from practice and other clinical records.
● The *ability* to benefit does not mean that every outcome will be favourable. Outcomes can only be known after the event but the need must be assessed beforehand.
● The *benefit* is not just a question of clinical status but includes all outcomes of relevance to the patient including reassurance, relief of carers, and supportive care.
● Health *care* includes not just treatment but also pre-

vention, diagnosis, continuing care, rehabilitation and palliative care.

Because need is the population's ability to benefit, it obviously depends on the *numbers* of people involved, and on there being an *intervention* that works. In short, interventions which do no good at all are not needed.

PRINCIPLES OF EPIDEMIOLOGICALLY BASED NEEDS ASSESSMENT

These are as follows:

● Needs are best recognized in terms of people with a specific disease rather than some other characteristic (such as age) or some other starting point such as arbitrary service boundaries. The reason is that a need arises when something has gone wrong rather than because a person has reached the age of 65 years or is served by a particular provider. Because many diseases affect a wide spectrum of patients it is often necessary to consider patient subcategories. For example, in the case of coronary heart disease the needs of the population as a whole, those with stable angina and those who have had a recent infarction are not the same.*
● Need is specifically distinguished from demand and supply although all three overlap (see Fig. 1.2, p. 5)., and to some extent it is the purchaser's role to try to maximize the overlap between the fields.

The distinction between need and supply, although theoretically obvious, is sometimes forgotten when needs assessment is information (i.e. current activity) led. The distinction between need and demand is frequently ignored when patient preference information is easier to gather than research benefit data.

● Population needs depend on *both* numbers of people in the population with a particular disease (subcategory) *and* whether or not something can be done about it. The degree to which a patient may gain from being treated reflects their need.
● Needs are worth assessing when something is going to be done about the need. But there is no point in doing anything about the need if the need is already met. Hence there is always an assumption that baseline services, i.e. current provision, are known.

---

* Full subcategories of coronary heart disease:

I   Population as a whole
II   Population with high risk
III People with mild angina (International Classification of diseases (ICD) 413)
IV   People with severe angina (ICD 413)
V   People with myocardial infarction (ICD 410)
VI   People with long-term sequelae of coronary heart disease (ICD 411 and 414).

Epidemiologically based needs assessment, therefore, includes a statement of local service provision.

In short, the epidemiologically based needs assessment method is one of triangulation, as shown in Figure 6.1.

Prevalence and incidence

The prevalence (in chronic disease) or incidence (in acute disease) is always important in service planning, but is not the same as 'need'. Need depends on both numbers and effectiveness. Prevalence or incidence can only quantify unmet need where the known effectiveness of an established service is different from the potential caseload. There are many examples of this, including for example *end-stage renal failure,* where any deficit in provision below the incidence of the condition should raise questions about unmet need. Similarly, the prevalence of *severe dementia* will give a good clue as to the levels of service (even if not the details) that may be required. What such widely different disease groups have in common is at least an assumption that something useful can be done. In end-stage renal failure, renal replacement therapy is life-saving. In severe dementia, relieving the burden of informal carers is a benefit, whether or not the patients are acknowledged by the health services.

The main problem in assessing incidence and prevalence is the poverty of suitable data. However, the data are seldom absent altogether. There are three major sources – national routine data, local data and research data. Whatever the shortcomings of each of these individually, collectively they are often useful. Research data do not have to be local. For example, the incidence of *stroke* in Oxfordshire (Bamford et al, 1988, 1990) is not greatly different from the incidence of stroke elsewhere in southern England, and the degree to which it differs between southern and northern England or Scotland is reasonably well known. Service planning is still possible.

But such data as are gathered from various heterogeneous sources should be used with caution. Caution should concern the following questions:

1. Are the data collected accurately? This is a special problem with hospital records, for example.

2. Are the data about the same patients I am interested in? Patients with the same disease are often drawn from quite different population groups, i.e. patients presenting to a teaching hospital may be much more severely ill with a disease than those with an identical label asking their pharmacist for advice. Again with the stroke example, clearly the requirements of someone who is hemiplegic are quite different from those of someone who has had a stroke lasting barely longer than a transient ischaemic attack.

3. Are the data applicable here? Clearly some diseases vary widely in their incidence and prevalence – notably infectious diseases. The incidence of AIDS in the northwest quadrant of London is quite different from the incidence of AIDS in rural Devon. This, however, should not be an excuse to ignore the data altogether.

4. Are the data applicable reliably to small samples? Although the incidence of myocardial infarction can be reliably guessed for a health authority covering 0.5 million people, it will be notoriously pulsatile in a single general practice. Indeed, diagnostic rates for most conditions are so low as to be very unpredictable at practice levels. A general practitioner will only see one case of new thyroid cancer every 25 years and even only one new case of lung cancer every year (on average) (Fry 1993). The more services that are planned at an aggregated level, the less of a problem this is. If the prevalence of a condition is less than 1% it would be unwise to estimate numbers at a single practice level. Epidemiological rates should be used for guidance only.

Effectiveness (and cost-effectiveness) of services

Perhaps the main problem of working with incidence and prevalence data is that they have very little meaning if there is significant uncertainty about whether current interventions are really beneficial. The prevalence of the common cold says very little about the need for consultations in primary care, secondary care or anywhere else. There is clearly no point recruiting patients who have a self-limiting disease for which there is no treatment. This is the converse of the end-stage renal failure example. The effectiveness of health services is increasingly recognized as a central domain for NHS research. However, initiatives to sort out effectiveness

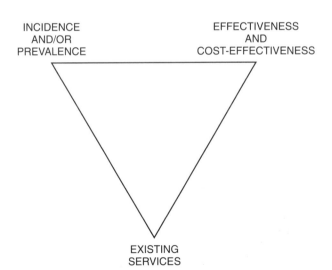

Figure 6.1   A graphic illustration of the epidemiologically based needs assessment method.

do not have a long history, and many interventions are of doubtful effectiveness. Perhaps the main task from the point of view of both district health authorities and GPs as purchasers, is the gathering together of the evidence on what works and what does not. However, there are a number of initiatives bringing this information to purchasers in accessible forms. 'Systematic reviews' are increasingly being produced by health service researchers summarizing the evidence on the effectiveness of different interventions. For example, the national roles of the UK Cochrane Centre, and the NHS Centre for Reviews and Dissemination (Sheldon & Chalmers 1994) and the regional role of the South and West Development and Evaluation Committee (Stevens 1993, 1994, 1995), The *Health Care Needs Assessment* series (Stevens and Raftery 1994) attempts to pull together the effectiveness information on each of the 20 diseases it deals with.

Knowledge of what works and what does not work in health care offers perhaps the greatest current scope for changing health services to meet needs. The arguably over-provided routine child health care screening is more than matched by, say, the under-provision of antiplatelet prophylaxis after stroke and myocardial infarction. Examples of under-provided effective interventions and over-provided ineffective provisions abound, in the sources described above and elsewhere, e.g. *Bandolier* (Moore et al 1995).

What should one do in practice if the evidence is unclear? There is seldom no evidence whatsoever. Evidence can be graded by its quality, and there are a number of schemes for doing this such as the one in Table 6.1 adapted from the US Preventive Services Task Force (1989).

The decision on how much change to call for where the evidence is weak can be made pragmatically. If all other things are equal, there are plenty of areas in health care where the evidence is strong and the costs of making change are not unreasonable which should be given priority. Equally, with new interventions where there may be pressure to adopt them but the evidence is weak, e.g. the use of expensive new drugs with limited patient benefit (e.g. DNase in cystic fibrosis), it is probably worth resisting vast expenditure (Robert 1994) because of the opportunity cost of the resources.

Existing services

Despite the paucity of information on incidence and prevalence and effectiveness, ironically the most difficult information sometimes to get hold of is the baseline of existing services. Within primary care, of course, the GP is in a strong position to know what services are provided. In secondary care such information needs to be

Table 6.1 Quality and force of research evidence on effectiveness

Quality of the evidence[a]

I	Evidence obtained from at least one properly randomized controlled trial
II–1	Evidence obtained from well-designed controlled trials without randomization
II–2	Evidence obtained from well-designed cohort or case-control analytical studies, preferably from more than one centre or research group
II–3	Evidence obtained from multiple timed series with or without the intervention, or from dramatic results in uncontrolled experiments
III	Opinions of respected authorities based on clinical experience, descriptive studies or reports of expert committees
IV	Evidence inadequate owing to problems of methodology, e.g. sample size, length or comprehensiveness of follow-up, or conflict in evidence

Strength of recommendation

A	There is good reason to support the use of the procedure
B	There is fair reason to support the use of the procedure
C	There is poor reason to support the use of the procedure
D	There is fair reason to reject the use of the procedure
E	There is good reason to support the rejection of the use of the procedure

[a]Such evidence grades should be accompanied by a note on the strength of the recommendation (based on the cost-effectiveness of the procedure as shown in the second part of the table).

carefully extracted from providers. Ideally one would know the quantity, quality and unit cost of the services. For example, in the case of end-stage renal failure services a health commission should wish to know the total quality of all the renal replacement modalities set out in Table 6.2 (see p. 76); similarly for a consortium of GPs, but an individual GP might be satisfied just knowing about availability and relative cost of the alternatives without the need to know total supply. Similarly in *alcohol services* the service headings to be aware of might be as shown in Box 6.1.

Box 6.1 Alcohol services baseline check-list

Prevention
- Health promotion
- Local action on prevention

Generic social services
- Statutory social services (number of specialist social workers)
- Non-statutory social services

GP and primary health care
- GP and primary health care (early detection and simple interventions)

NHS non-specialist hospital services
- General (non-psychiatric) hospital services (e.g. joint clinics, alcohol misuse screening)
- General district psychiatric services

Specialist services for alcohol misuse
- Specialized NHS treatment services
- Liaison team (i.e. community alcohol team)
- Private health care organizations

PRACTICAL USE OF EPIDEMIOLOGICAL NEEDS ASSESSMENT IN PRIMARY CARE

How in practice can the epidemiological approach to needs assessment be used in primary care? What difficulties may arise? How can it help primary care teams who may already feel overwhelmed by their workload?

Three scenarios will be considered:

1. Primary care as purchasers
2. Primary care as providers
3. Primary care as both purchasers and providers.

Primary care as purchasers

Where primary care teams are acting as purchasers, it will often not be necessary or desirable for them to perform the entire assessment of need for each condition of interest personally. There is still a dearth of easily available information on prevalence and effectiveness, and that which is available has an inherent bias towards secondary care. Much of the evidence in the secondary care field is complex, requiring familiarity with epidemiology, statistics, critical appraisal and economic evaluation. Such familiarity is more likely in units where such work is concentrated, such as academic departments of public health medicine. In addition, the numbers of patients affected in individual practices are often too small, and repeating the exercise in different commissioning groups is inefficient. It may thus be more sensible for primary care teams to adapt epidemiologically based needs assessments produced on either a regional or national basis in these circumstances.

Conditions where effectiveness is uncertain

In the South and West region ('Wessex'), the principles of epidemiological needs assessment have been applied to a number of new 'technologies' (including drugs, devices, procedures and settings) (Stevens 1993, 1994, 1995), where the principal question is one of effectiveness. The resulting reports are published, and assist commissioners (including general practitioners) in deciding whether to purchase the technology. Box 6.2 briefly considers *serum screening for Down's syndrome** as an example, to inform purchasers whose patients are not serum screened (and perhaps even where they are) whether there is a need for serum screening as opposed to age-based selection for amniocentesis (Sadler 1994).

Such evidence simplifies the evidence for purchasers, and can also be used to provide information to patients, potentially giving greater choice to women.

* Produced for the South and West Development and Evaluation Committee (the 'Wessex' DEC at the time of the Down's screening report).

Box 6.2   Serum screening for Down's syndrome – an adaptation of epidemiologically based needs assessment

Prevalence in Wessex (population 3 million)
- 33 000 deliveries per year
- 180 cases of Down's syndrome per year

Current service
- Amniocentesis based on maternal age (1200)
- Detection rate 27.5%
- Prevents 10 cases of Down's syndrome per year (based on 66% survival to term in the absence of termination and 90% termination rate)

Effectiveness and cost of serum screening
- Detection rate between 37.5 and 65% (equivalent to between 7 and 23 *additional* cases detected per year)
- Prevents an *additional* 4–13 cases per year (based on 66% survival to term in the absence of termination and 90% termination rate)
- Will require more amniocenteses, and thus cause loss of more normal fetuses (between 1 and 4 *additional* losses per year)
- Other disbenefits
- Will cost up to £1.2 million to introduce
- Marginal cost per additional case detected of between £57 000 and £176 000

Conditions where effectiveness is known, but the numbers requiring the intervention are not

An example of the use of epidemiological needs assessment in these circumstances is provided by *end-stage renal failure*. Renal replacement therapy (RRT), either by dialysis or transplantation, is highly effective in providing a good quality of life in an otherwise inevitably fatal condition. Transplantation is the most effective treatment modality, both in terms of cost and the quality and duration of survival (Beech et al 1994), but is limited by the relative lack of donor organs.

The 1994 UK acceptance rate for RRT in the UK was 65 patients per million of the population, which is lower than most other countries in the Western world, and lower than the best estimate of population need in the UK. The overall incidence of end-stage renal failure suitable for RRT, in those aged less than 80 years, is 78 per million of the population per year. The prevalence of end-stage renal failure is almost the same as the prevalence of patients receiving RRT (stock), and an acceptance rate of 78 per million would lead to a 'steady state' stock of 800 per million. Thus, in a practice with 10 000 patients, one would expect eight patients on RRT. The number is likely to vary with the age and ethnic structure of the practice population (as well as with chance), the incidence of ESRF increasing with age and being higher in people of Asian or Afro-Caribbean origin.

Rationing of RRT has been largely covert, GPs, hospital physicians and surgeons often not referring patients to nephrologists for assessment when they might have benefitted (Beech et al 1994). Estimates of population need, together with assessment of current services, will allow primary care teams to assess whether they are likely to have unrecognized or unmet need (Box 6.3).

Box 6.3 Do current services meet healthcare needs?

- Have all those with the condition been identified?
- Have all those identified received the interventions that are known to be effective?

The likely costs of purchasing services for end-stage renal failure can also be estimated (Table 6.2).

Table 6.2 Costs of renal replacement therapy

Treatment modality	Percentage of stock	Annual NHS cost (1990 prices)
Hospital haemodialysis	17	£18 000
Home haemodialysis	6	£11 000
CAPD	22	£13 000
Kidney transplant	55	£10 000 (operation) – year 1 £3 000 (maintenance) – subsequent years

CAPD, continuous ambulatory peritoneal dialysis.

Primary care as providers

The triangulation principle may be very easily applied to the provision of primary care, and can facilitate service planning as primary care widens its scope beyond a demand-led service. In these circumstances, the needs assessment is best carried out by the primary care team itself, as not only will much of the data be available within the practice, but the individuality of primary care provision militates against the assessment being performed by centrally based academic units.

The central principles of epidemiologically based needs assessment remain the same; the first question is whether the treatment or service works, and the second is how many people can benefit. Two detailed practical examples of the application of these methods in general practice to specific clinical areas will be considered. They form part of a project on health care needs assessment which is being carried out jointly by the Portsmouth and South East Hampshire Health Commission and one non-fundholding practice in the Commission area (Box 6.4). The first example looks at interventions for patients with a previous myocardial infarction, and is worked up in some detail to demonstrate the process. The second covers a less well-defined area, that of alcohol misuse, and demonstrates some of the potential pitfalls in carrying out this form of assessment. It should be noted that both examples are subcategories of wider clinical areas, i.e. coronary heart disease and excess alcohol intake, respectively. Such subcategorization is a crucial step in needs assessment, and will be considered further later in this chapter.

Box 6.4 Epidemiologically based needs assessment in primary care in Portsmouth

The practice
- Four partners
- 7839 patients
- Suburban

The conditions
- Secondary prevention following myocardial infarction
- Alcohol misuse

Carrying out an epidemiological needs assessment in primary care

Process. The process is as follows:

1. *Choose the condition(s)* (Box 6.5). Sources of evidence on effectiveness are dealt with elsewhere in this book (see Ch. 12), but the *Health Care Needs Assessment* series (Stevens & Raftery 1994) which deals with 20 conditions, including both of these examples, is a good starting point.

Box 6.5 Choosing the condition(s) for which to assess need

Essential
- Can be clearly defined
- Interventions for which there is reasonable evidence of effectiveness/ineffectiveness*
- Reasonable data on occurrence (epidemiology)

Preferable
- Condition of interest to primary care team
- Manageable number of cases (will depend on staffing and information technology)
- Information on current service easily available (e.g. by audit of primary care notes)

* Needs assessment may also be used to assess whether there is 'overmet' need for conditions where care is ineffective, e.g. screening for prostate cancer, dilatation and curettage in women under 40 years of age.

---

2. *Derive indicative prevalence for the practice.* The data from published sources, national or local, are applied to the practice population to calculate an expected number of cases for the practice. This may be performed crudely by multiplying the population prevalence by the practice population. (For epilepsy, for example: prevalence of active epilepsy is 0.5% (Manford 1992); practice population is 7850; expected numbers are 7850 × 0.05 = 39.) In conditions where the prevalence varies more with age and sex, the age–sex-specific prevalence from the published data should be multiplied by the numbers in the relevant age–sex band in the practice. Table 6.3 sets this out for previous myocardial infarction patients.

Clearly, figures derived from one population will not necessarily apply in a different part of the country, e.g. where the socioeconomic composition differs from the average; and there are bound to be local variations because of small numbers. However, the derived figures

Table 6.3 Indicative prevalence of previous myocardial infarction (MI) in males in the practice population

Age band (years)	No. of males in the age band in the practice	Prevalence (%)	Expected numbers with previous MI
35–39	300	0.5	1
40–44	290	1.7	5
45–49	290	3.3	10
50–54	290	5.2	15
55–59	220	6.6	13
60–64	120	7.0	8
65–74[a]	190	10.5	20
75–84[a]	100	7.0	7
85+	15	5.0	1
Total			80

Sources: Shaper (1984) and OPCS (1994).
[a]10 year age bands.

will provide an *indication* of the numbers that might be expected in the practice.

3. *Produce a brief summary of effective interventions.* Box 6.6 summarizes a list of interventions for *previous myocardial infarction* that can be performed in primary care, for which there is good evidence of effectiveness (Dunnigan 1993, Sever et al 1993, Flapan 1994, Langham et al 1994, Pyorala et al 1994). Use of angiotensin-converting enzyme (ACE) inhibitors in patients with left ventricular impairment could be added, though may require secondary care input for assessment.

All the interventions in Box 6.6 would be classified as AI or AII (see Table 6.1), i.e. strongly recommended and based on good trial data. Having calculated the expected numbers of relevant patients and having identified the most valuable interventions, the next step is to compare this with the patients known to the practice.

Box 6.6 Effective interventions in patients with previous myocardial infarction

- Recent (within past 12 months) smoking status should be recorded, and advice on cessation provided
- At least one measurement of blood cholesterol, taken after the infarct, should be recorded. Blood cholesterol above 5.5 mmol/l should be treated, by diet for 6 months, and then by cholesterol-lowering treatment if the level remains above 5.5 mmol/l
- First-degree relatives of any patient suffering from a myocardial infarction before the age of 50 years should have their cholesterol level measured, and their cardiovascular risk assessed
- Blood pressure should be measured at least annually, and diastolic pressure maintained below 90 mmHg
- Patients should be on aspirin 75–325 mg/day unless specifically contraindicated
- Patients should be on a β blocker unless specifically contraindicated

---

4. *Search practice records* (Box 6.7).

Box 6.7 Search strategy for patients with previous myocardial infarction

- **Read codes on computerized medical summary:**
  - G30/G32 are the main diagnostic codes
  - 14A3/14A4 (history of myocardial infarction)
  - 323 (myocardial infarction on ECG)
- **Coronary heart disease register** (required for band 3 health promotion programme)
- **All those on low-dose aspirin**
- **Word of mouth** – partners, district nurses, etc.

---

5. *Audit records of identified patients to see if effective interventions have been applied.* This would ideally require a systematic inspection of records, but could in theory be undertaken opportunistically by flagging records and interviewing when the patients visit for other reasons.

6. *Assess unmet need**:

a. The number of patients with the condition that are unknown to the practice (as indicated by a difference in the numbers identified in the practice from the calculated indicative prevalence).

b. The number of patients known to the practice who are not receiving all of the effective interventions.

Similar principles may be applied to needs assessment for *alcohol misuse* (Box 6.8). The evidence is taken from Edwards & Unnithal (1994) and Freemantle et al (1993). This example is chosen because this is an important problem in primary care, affecting several hundred patients, and there is strong evidence of the effectiveness of a simple and inexpensive intervention, but the process of needs assessment may not be straightforward. The main problem lies in the assessment of the current service. This relates to three separate issues:

1. *Definition.* The stated definition excludes those drinking above these levels who have either problems or dependence. In practice, the search strategy is unlikely to be able to exclude these patients. Inclusion of all drinkers above this level increases the potential numbers markedly (prevalence of 25% of males and 11% of females). In addition, though brief intervention may be helpful in those with problems or dependence, other forms of more intensive treatment will be required by others.

2. *Search.* Unlike myocardial infarction, alcohol misuse is unlikely to be mentioned on a hospital discharge summary, or, in the absence of problems or dependence, to have merited a note in the summary of medical history. The information will thus need to be obtained from the health promotion data for the majority of patients. Such

---

* In theory the same applies to 'overmet need', i.e. unnecessary interventions of no benefit.

Box 6.8 Epidemiological needs assessment for alcohol misuse (without problems or dependence, i.e. category I from Edwards & Unnithal (1994)) (the other two categories are 'excessive drinking with problems but without dependence' (II) and 'Excessive drinking with problems and dependence' (III))

Definition
- Excessive drinking (>21 units per week for men, >14 units per week for women) without problems or dependence

Read codes
- E250 main diagnostic code
- EMIS input code Egton 418 (this code will vary, depending on the system used by the practice) – search for >21 in males, >14 in females
- 136 (alcohol consumption)
- 6892 (alcohol consumption screen)

Search strategy
- Health promotion data under Egton 418
- Read codes under computerized medical summary

Expected numbers
- Prevalence for persons aged 18 years or over: 13% in males, 7% in females. Application of these percentages to the practice population produces an indicative prevalence of 360 males and 204 females in this practice

Effective intervention
- Brief intervention in primary care, consisting of assessment of intake, and provision of information and advice, produces a fall of over 20% in alcohol consumption
- Costs around £20 per patient

---

data may not be available for many of the practice population. Even where recorded, it may not be accurate. Patients may deliberately or accidentally underestimate consumption, and recorded values may not be exact where alcohol consumption is merely one of several values being noted rather than a central reason for the visit. One strategy would be to start to record the information prospectively as a deliberate needs assessment policy.

3. *Interventions.* The provision of advice and information specifically relating to alcohol intake may not be recorded where consumption is noted as part of a battery of questions on lifestyle.

Impact. The potential pitfalls discussed above do not mean that epidemiologically based needs assessment is not useful in alcohol misuse. They are merely pointers to consider before embarking on such assessment within a practice.

This project is still ongoing, and therefore we cannot fully quantify the final costs and impact. However, it has already provided direction to the programme of audit within the practice, and demonstrated the deficiencies in the practices' computerized records, not only in the completeness of data, but also in the interpretation and use of the data available.

Primary care as both purchasers and providers

For many conditions, primary care will be both providing

care, and commissioning or purchasing care. *Coronary heart disease* is a good example, and is a key area in Health of the Nation. Consideration of this clinical area will illustrate how the application of epidemiologically based needs assessment in primary care may assist in setting priorities for intervention. Coronary heart disease accounts for over one-quarter of all deaths in the UK, and is a significant cause of premature mortality. The majority of general practices collected data on the risk factors for coronary heart disease through their participation in the former Health Promotion banding scheme. How can primary care teams provide and purchase services that will reduce the burden of coronary heart disease?

Prevalence – sources of information

A practice that was registered for Band 3 of the Health Promotion programme will have a register of patients with hypertension and coronary heart disease, and will have collected information on smoking, body mass index and family history in those aged 15–74 years.

A list of 'indicative prevalences', for a practice of 10 000 patients, for coronary heart disease and many of the associated risk factors has also been produced (Charlton et al 1994). These can be used for comparison with the practice data, or alone where practice data are unavailable. Box 6.9 shows the risk factors for which information may be available.

Box 6.9 Available information on prevalence of coronary heart disease and associated risk factors at practice level

Primary prevention
- Smoking
- Hypertension
- Obesity
- Exercise
- Family history

Secondary prevention
- Angina
- Previous myocardial infarction

Effectiveness of interventions

The effectiveness of an intervention to reduce coronary heart disease relates not only to the ability of that intervention to modify the risk factor, but also the importance of the risk factor in the aetiology of disease, and the feasibility of applying the intervention to the at-risk population. Table 6.4 indicates those interventions where there is strong evidence of the effectiveness of intervention in primary care (modified from Langham et al 1994), and an indication of the numbers likely to be involved in a practice of 10 000 (Charlton et al 1994). Table 6.5 indicates those interventions where there is strong evidence of the

Table 6.4 Effective primary care interventions in coronary heart disease

Risk factor	No. in practice with 10 000 patients	Intervention
Smoking	2 700	Cessation advice and support
Hypertension	1 150	Identification and treatment
Angina/previous myocardial infarction	500	Aspirin, β blockers, ACE inhibitors, advice on cessation of smoking, control of hypertension and hypercholesterolaemia

Table 6.5 Effective secondary care interventions in coronary heart disease

Risk factor	No. in practice with 10 000 patients	Intervention
Myocardial infarction	25 per year	Early thrombolysis
Left main coronary artery disease/three vessel disease	3 per year[a]	Coronary artery bypass grafting

[a] This figure reflects the current supply. The level of need for coronary artery bypass grafting, as defined by ability to benefit, remains a matter of debate. This figure is used to indicate the likely order of need.

effectiveness of intervention in secondary care, again with an indication of the likely numbers.

Effective secondary care interventions in coronary heart disease. Tables 6.4 and 6.5 indicate that the vast majority of patients who have a health care need in relation to coronary heart disease should have that need met in primary care. They also demonstrate the importance of considering subcategories both of the disease area, and the population. Thus the nature and provider of the intervention, and the numbers able to benefit, depend on whether one is dealing with the whole practice population, those at high risk, or those with established coronary artery disease. The strength of the evidence, and the cost of intervention, also vary. There is good evidence that coronary artery bypass grafting is effective in the presence of left main coronary artery disease or three-vessel disease, but the evidence does not support coronary artery bypass grafting in patients without such extensive coronary artery disease. Table 6.6 shows the relative utility* of some alternative interventions for coronary heart disease (Langham et al 1994).

Such data illustrate the relative cost-effectiveness of simple interventions that can be carried out in primary care, and may allow a comparison of purchasing options

*'Cost utility' differs from 'cost-effectiveness', in that it describes the benefits such that they may be compared between diseases, i.e. by using quality-adjusted life-years saved.

Table 6.6 Cost-utility of interventions in coronary heart disease in terms of cost per quality-adjusted life years (QALY) gained (1990 prices)

Intervention	Extra cost per QALY gained
GP advice to stop smoking	£200
Pacemaker for heart block	£850
CABG for severe angina and left main artery disease	£1 300
Heart transplantation	£6 100
CABG for mild angina and two-vessel disease	£16 300

CABG, coronary artery bypass grafting.

across different clinical areas as cost-utility approaches become more widespread.

Current services

Assessment of the current services can again be performed by comparing the numbers known to the practice with the indicative prevalence; and then checking the records to see whether the effective interventions are being applied. This will indicate the extent to which patient's healthcare needs are being met, and enable attention to be focused on any shortfall or over-provision identified.

CONCLUSION

Boxes 6.10 and 6.11 summarize the advantages and disadvantages of the epidemiological method of needs assessment in primary care.

It is unlikely that any needs assessment will be flawless. What is more important is that it should lead to consideration of the ways of identifying and treating patients who could benefit from health care. Epidemiologically based needs assessment offers one means of achieving this, particularly when strategic resource shifts or new service developments are proposed.

Box 6.10 Advantages of the epidemiological method of needs assessment in primary care

- It enables an assessment of health care need
- It enables an assessment of unmet need
- It is based on nationally researched and published data, providing uniformity, but can be applied to individual practices with different standards of data collection
- Assessment of need can encompass interventions at both primary and secondary care level
- It brings together the complementary skills of public health and primary care practitioners
- It can facilitate the introduction and auditing of guidelines into primary care
- The method can be applied on any condition for which there is published evidence on epidemiology and the effectiveness of interventions, and by any number of practices in a district

---

Box 6.11 Disadvantages of epidemiological method of needs assessment in primary care

- To be worth doing, it must be done properly, requiring commitment of time of public health specialists, as well as the expense of training practice staff
- Available information on epidemiology and effectiveness mainly available only for secondary care at present
- The available data may not accurately reflect the local picture
- The method treats the incorporation of patient opinion as a separate activity
- Individual practices may only have small numbers of patients with conditions of interest, making interpretation of data unreliable
- The searching for information, especially of notes to assess compliance with standards, takes a lot of time. The amount of time will depend on the state of the records in the practice

---

REFERENCES

Bamford J, Sandercock P, Dennis M et al 1988 A prospective study of acute cerebrovascular disease in the community: the Oxfordshire Community Stroke Project. 1. Methodology, demography and incident cases of first-ever stroke. Journal of Neurology, Neurosurgery and Psychiatry 51: 1373–1380

Bamford J, Sandercock P, Dennis M, Warlow C 1990 A prospective study of acute cerebrovascular disease in the community: The Oxfordshire Community Stroke Project. 2. Incidence, case fatality rates and overall outcome at one year of cerebral infarction, primary intracerebral and subarachnoid haemorrhage. Journal of Neurology and Psychiatry 53: 16–22

Beech R, Gulliford M, Mays N, Melia J, Roderick P 1994 Renal disease. In: Stevens A, Raftery J (eds) Health care needs assessment. Radcliffe Medical Press, Oxford, pp. 58–110

Charlton B G, Calvert N, White M, Rye G, Conrad W, van Zwanenberg T 1994 Health promotion priorities for general practice: constructing and using 'indicative prevalences'. British Medical Journal 308: 1019–1022

Dunnigan M 1993 The problem with cholesterol. British Medical Journal 306: 1355–1356

Edwards G, Unnithal S 1994 Alcohol misuse. In: Stevens A, Raftery J (eds) Health care needs assessment. Radcliffe Medical Press, Oxford, pp. 341–374

Flapan A 1994 Management of patients after their first myocardial infarction. British Medical Journal 309: 1129–1134

Freemantle N, Gill P, Godfrey C et al 1993 Brief interventions and alcohol use – are brief interventions effective in reducing harm associated with alcohol consumption? Effective Health Care 7

Fry J 1993 General practice: the facts. NAHAT, Radcliffe Medical Press, Oxford

Langham S, Normand C, Piercy J, Rose G 1994 Coronary heart disease. In: Stevens A, Raftery J (eds) Health care needs assessment. Radcliffe Medical Press, Oxford, pp. 341–375

Manford M 1992 Treatment of epilepsy. The Practitioner 236: 984–987

Moore A, McQuay H, Gray M 1995 Bandolier – the first 20 issues. Classic Press, Oxford

Morbidity Statistics for General Practice 1991/2. 1994 OPCS

Pyorala K, De Backer G, Poole-Wilson P, Wood D 1994 Prevention of coronary heart disease in clinical practice. Recommendations of the task force of the European Society of Cardiology, European Atherosclerosis Society and European Society of Hypertension. European Heart Journal 15: 1300–1331

Robert G 1994 Recombinant Human DNase for cystic fibrosis. In: Stevens A (ed) Health technology evaluation research reviews. Wessex Institute of Public Health Medicine, Winchester

Sadler M 1994 Serum screening for Down's syndrome. In: Stevens A (ed) Health technology evaluation research reviews. Wessex Institute of Public Health Medicine, Winchester

Sever P, Beevers G, Bulpitt C, Lever A, Ramsay L, Reid J, Swales J 1993 Management guidelines in essential hypertension; report of the second working party of the British Hypertension Society. British Medical Journal 306: 983–987

Shaper A, Cook D, Walker M, Macfarlane P 1984 Prevalence of ischaemic heart disease in middle aged British men. British Heart Journal 51: 595–605

Sheldon T, Chalmers I 1994 The Cochrane Centre and the NHS Centre for Reviews and Dissemination: respective roles within the Information Systems Strategy of the NHS R&D Programme, coordination and principles underlying collaboration. Health Economics 32: 201–203

Stevens A (ed) 1993 Health technology evaluation research reviews. Wessex Institute of Public Health Medicine, 209 pp

Stevens A (ed) 1994 Health technology evaluation research reviews. Wessex Institute of Public Health Medicine, 242 pp

Stevens A (ed) 1995 Health technology evaluation research reviews. Wessex Institute of Public Health Medicine, 249 pp

Stevens A, Raftery J (eds) 1994 Health care needs assessment. Radcliffe Medical Press, Oxford

US Preventive Services Task Force 1989 Guide to clinical preventive services. An assessment of the effectiveness of 169 interventions. Williams and Wilkins, Baltimore

7

Needs assessment for fundholders

Valerie Chisty

The provision for general practitioners (GPs) to become fundholders was one of the key tenets of the National Health Service (NHS) reforms. The fund comprises three elements – a budget for a range of hospital and community health services, a cash-limited drugs budget, and a budget for staff. Since the concept was introduced in 1991, various changes have been made both to the entry criteria and to the range of services included within the fund. There are presently two levels of fundholding available to GPs – standard and community fundholding – and a third option of 'total purchasing'.

The concept of fundholding has introduced greater flexibility for GPs, with regard to the contractual arrangements which they make, the opportunity to make savings and to vire resources between the different fund headings (i.e. transfer funds from one budget to another, e.g. drugs to staff) in order to develop new services or extend existing health care. Virement opportunities also exist across the primary/secondary care interface, and examples of shifts exist in both directions, e.g. purchasing additional hospital activity to reduce waiting lists, and reducing outpatient activity with further follow-up in primary care. This concept is stretched further with total purchasing, where GPs hold devolved responsibility for the entire range of care for their patients, rather than the limited list within fundholding. The most significant difference between fundholding and total purchasing is the responsibility for purchasing emergency care, and the extent of risk and unpredictability which this introduces.

Fundholding has focused thinking on the role of the GP in needs assessment, but needs assessment at the practice level should be seen as integral to the primary care-led NHS, regardless of the technical mechanisms for organizing resources. All GPs, whether total purchasers, fundholders or nonfundholders, commit resources in terms of enabling patients to access care and treatment. Within fundholding and total purchasing, the resources become transparent, and GPs are made aware of the costs of care and the extent of the budget available. This brings GPs face to face with the potentially competing needs of the individual compared with the population. Some GPs have actively responded to this need to manage the funds and define priorities. Needs assessment can provide an objective way in which the health status of the practice population be determined and the competing demands for care can be prioritized.

This chapter describes examples of how fundholding practices are seeking to base purchasing decisions on a sound assessment of health need. The implications and lessons learnt from these examples will be explored and conclusions drawn.

EXAMPLE 1. HEALTH NEEDS ASSESSMENT AT THE HADLEIGH PRACTICE
Dr C. J. McCall, The Hadleigh Practice, Bournemouth, Dorset

Objectives

The Hadleigh Practice became a fundholder in April 1992, driven by the belief that the scheme would provide the means to maintain or improve standards of service delivery to patients. The objective of the practice was to establish formal means of assessing the health needs and health experience of their patients, rather than relying on perceptions, anecdotes and single events. The practice approached the needs of patients from the aspects of activity and quality, recognizing that, while fundholding forces an urgency in ensuring that contracts for activity are in place, quality aspects are equally important.

Process

Activity assessment for contract setting

Hadleigh had long collected data regarding the incidence of disease, originally paper based and more recently in computerized form, in order to create morbidity registers. While the logging of every referral letter which left the practice enabled identification of the demand placed on hospitals, information on the outcome of referrals was lacking. The year preparing for fundholding was used to begin to track referrals and gather information on the quantity and quality of activity. This process has been facilitated by fundholding, in which systems for tracking episodes of care through invoices and clinical summaries are adopted. The accumulation of data through the years has enabled the practice to develop a spreadsheet for monitoring all referrals and contract activity which forms the baseline for needs assessment. This enables cumulative monthly trends to be plotted in order to predict activity levels for common procedures, and estimate the contingency sums needed for the accumulation of rare events, which, while diffi-

cult to anticipate in isolation from one year to the next, can be predicted in aggregation.

Quality assessment for contract setting

The practice decided to address the issue of quality from the aspect of the patient, by identifying what the patients expect and receive. This approach was in accordance with that of the local health authority, which had undertaken a consultation exercise on aspects of quality as well as fundholding colleagues.

From an early stage, 'exit monitoring' questionnaires were introduced for patients who attended hospital outpatients departments, accident and emergency, or had an inpatient or day-case procedure (Box 7.1). The information obtained was analysed, and reports produced to assess useful aspects of quality which are important to the patient, as well as supporting contract monitoring.

Box 7.1   Example of an exit monitoring tool for planned admissions
Expected date of admission? ....   Was this cancelled by the hospital? Yes/no   If so, what was the date you heard? ....   Were you told why? Yes/no   Were you given another date at the time? Yes/no   Actual date of admission? ....   Date of discharge (even if same date)? ....   How much notice of discharge were you given? ....   If you needed to take medication home, did   you receive this promptly? Yes/no   Were you given a letter for your GP? Yes/no

Using data to inform contract specifications

Specific activities undertaken within the practice can also be used to inform needs assessment. For example, health checks for the over 75 year olds are undertaken by a designated community nurse who records her findings on a pro forma in the patients' notes and enters on the computer that the check has taken place. Patients can then be identified from the computer database and analysis undertaken to gather information such as chiropody contacts and use of walking aids. The acceptability of proposals by the local trust to change the method of delivering chiropody services was measured against the practice knowledge of patients needs.

Using patient experience to improve quality

Occasionally, aspects of care are identified which appear to the health professionals to be in need of change but where simple methods of achieving improved outcomes are not feasible. In such situations, a modified form of the 'focus group' has been employed to enable patient consultation to inform the planning process. From the disease morbidity database, patients (or their carers) who have the relevant condition have been identified, and invited to a meeting. Initially they are asked for their experiences and views of the current service, then their opinion on possible improvements, and their feedback on the practice proposals for change. Experience shows this to be an extremely productive mechanism for obtaining advice on the quality aspects of patients' needs.

Impact

1. No formal measurement of the impact of needs assessment has been undertaken, but it appears to have improved the quality of decision making in the practice, and the nature of contract monitoring. The assessments all continue.

2. The information on walking aids contributed to the development of a practice-based occupational therapist, part of whose remit is to assess the suitability of mobility aids for patients.

3. A greater involvement is being sought from the local public health department, whose knowledge of population-based health needs assessment will complement the practice's more individual patient-centred approach.

4. The practice also plans to explore a modified population health census, to enable comparisons with national estimates as well as answer specific local issues for the practice community.

EXAMPLE 2. INTO INFORMED PURCHASING – DISTRICT NURSING
G. Hewett, E. Brown and T. Evans,
Paxton Green Group Practice, London

Objectives

The Paxton Green Group Practice wished to commission district nursing services based on patient need, and decided to develop and test a model for needs assessment in order to commission primary care services at the practice level. The research task incorporated three objectives:

1. To identify the population's need for district nursing care
2. To identify need met by the existing service and to compare it with national and local statistics
3. To identify unmet need.

Process

The model (Hewett et al 1994) adopted a pragmatic approach to needs assessment, combining a quantitative study of activity data with qualitative interviews with local providers (both statutory and voluntary), users and carers.

The population's overall need was described by

examining sociodemographic characteristics from computerized records and local statistics. This information was augmented by interviews with 'local voices'. Data to describe met need were drawn from the West Lambeth Community Care (NHS) Trust's Comcare computer system and from manual records. The team's workload, case mix, primary activities and amount of time spent with patients was described and compared with national and local statistics. An analysis of unmet need was informed by the interview study, by published documents from the practice carers' group and an audit of need from the over 75 years olds' screening process. The study was undertaken by a part time researcher over 18 months, with research costs funded regionally.

Findings

Four key factors were found to influence the population's need for district nursing care:

- Clarity of the roles and relationships between the primary care nursing team, including the practice nurses, district nurses, health visitors and the nurse practitioner
- The culture of care at the practice which seeks to enable patients to remain at home
- Rising levels of deprivation
- The use and availability of other health and social care services, such as the increased use of day surgery and the availability of home helps.

The analysis of need showed:

- The existing team of 5.6 whole time equivalent district nurses was one whole time equivalent less than normally expected per 100 000 population
- The case load for the year under review averaged 97 clients per month, generating 8325 visits per annum
- Up to 65% of district nursing time was spent in face-to-face contact with patients – significantly higher than found in other studies.

Gaps and deficiencies in service were identified, and many of these overlapped with social care. These included a need for:

- Better information about services
- Greater provision of local day centres
- Wider availability of home-based respite care
- Agreed visiting times
- More time for counselling
- A laundry service for the incontinent
- Improved transport facilities for the disabled.

Impact and conclusions

1. It was possible to conduct a needs assessment study drawing principally on routinely collected and

locally derived information within an acceptable time-scale and budget.

2. To be fully effective, routinely collected data may need to be extended and tailored to the specific issue. For example, the information analysed enabled the identification of areas of unmet need plus a requirement for a larger district nursing team, but to inform purchasing decisions about the skill mix, additional details about patient dependency were required. Such measures of dependency must take into account the level of nursing skills necessary for each patient.

3. Recommendations incorporated within the contract included standardized recording of patient dependency scales which defined both nursing responsibilities and the dependency of the patient, as well as practical monitoring of patients' perceptions of quality, especially compliance with agreed visiting times.

4. The dependency tool was further developed by the nursing team and subsequently used in quarterly nursing case load monitoring.

5. Use of the tool confirmed the initial conclusions outlined above, resulting in the practice increasing investment in district nursing in the following year.

6. The dependency assessment tool has continued to be of value, forming the basis for agreeing contract activity in 1996–97, with the increased level of nursing being sustained. The concerns identified on laundry services and agreed visiting times have been addressed, and transport needs are being considered within a project being undertaken within the practice in 1996–97.

7. Some issues, however, are less amenable to practice-based solutions and can only be addressed by wider working with the health authority and social services.

EXAMPLE 3. SETTING PRIORITIES FOR REFERRALS

P. Ayres, Wakefield Health Authority

Objectives

Box 7.2   Aims and objectives

Aim
To develop an informed debate about 'value for money' in the context of the practice becoming fundholders.

Objectives
1. For sessions to be interactive
2. To explore the following areas:
   – The meaning of 'value for money'
   – Ethical issues
   – Potential role for health economics
3. To develop an implementation framework
4. To draw up a plan of action
5. To evaluate this series of workshops
6. To 'audit' the whole process in 1 year.

Process

The assignment took place as part of an experimental method of delivering public health advice to primary health care teams by placing a public health physician (PHP) in the surgeries of local GPs. The specific issue addressed was: *'development of the practice's definition of "value for money" in the context of fundholding'*.

A series of group discussion sessions was planned to address the key issues in priority planning for the practice. The subjects covered in each session are shown in Box 7.3. Nine interactive sessions took place, each lasting about 90 min. The whole project lasted for 6 months. The PHP was responsible for managing the production of documentation, and the timing and facilitation of the sessions. The group (made up of the PHP, all five partners in the practice and the practice manager) used much of the theoretical knowledge provided by the PHP in sessions 1–6 to formulate its own set of criteria (Table 7.1) for critically appraising referrals. The group also decided a system for applying the criteria in a process of managing/prioritizing referrals (Fig. 7.1) in a cash-limited position, which included having an 'appeals committee' which would formally consider competing referrals.

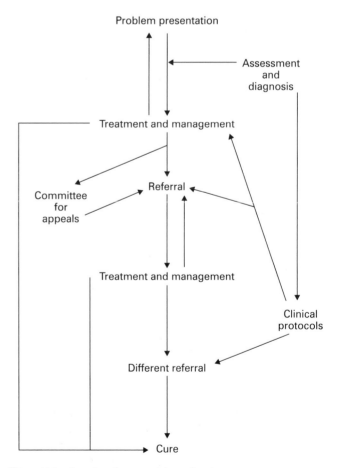

Figure 7.1   A system for appraising referrals.

Table 7.1 Criteria used for appraising referrals

Criteria	Weighting
1. Treatment factors:	
A. Effectiveness	50
B. Availability:	10
– locality	
– waiting lists	
C. Cost	10
2. Condition factors:	
A. Suffering	15
B. Health risk	15
	———
	100
3. Other factors (these may affect weighting either positively or	
negatively)	
A. Doctor:	
– coping with uncertainty	± 4
– level of knowledge	± 2
– heart sink	± 2
B. Patient:	
– stoicism (+)	± 3
– general condition	± 11
– expectation/demand	± 6

The success of this programme was mainly due to the following components:

- Commitment from the GPs and practice manager to 'make it work'
- Commitment from the PHP to allow the practice to take over the process
- Rigorous documentation of meetings and the outcomes of decision making
- Mutual respect of all participants – this allowed challenges to be considered openly and dealt with appropriately
- Sessions started and finished on time, and interruptions were kept to a minimum
- Attendance of the GPs at the meetings was seen by the whole group as mandatory, thus flexibility was needed to fit in with holidays, clinics, etc.

Impact

1. The practice incorporated the results of this work into the health planning processes for GP fundholding.

2. Auditing the whole process proved too arduous a task without information and technical support from the district health authority.

3. The group felt that having a referral system was a benefit drawn from this programme.

4. Other spin-offs which must happen in order to develop and run such a system included:
- Needing to discuss the reasons for interdoctor variation in referral behaviour
- Needing to discuss each other's value systems
- Working through difficult issues together
- Needing to access more information on effectiveness
- Planning strategies together for managing clinical problems.

Box 7.3 Content of the sessions

Session 1. Background to commissioning, agenda setting, timetable.

Session 2. Economic principles including:
- Definition of economics and scarcity
- The market
- The margin
- Economic evaluation techniques
- The Quality adjusted life years (QALY)
- Equity.

Session 3. Rationing healthcare: impact on the GP*
- Is there a need to ration?
- Rationing is already happening
- GPs do not want to ration 'face to face'
- The role of third party rationers
- How GPs can be included in third party decision-making processes

Session 4. Exploring 'value for money'
- Is effectiveness the 'be all and end all'?
- Should we compare treatments for different conditions?
- Should we try to be systematic in making prioritizing decisions?
- How do we decide when, and when not, to refer people for treatment?
- Is the practice's own definition of equity appropriate?
- Why do you (the practice) already offer the type of 'portfolio' of treatment to your patients which you do, and
- Why do you (the GP) refer some patients for some forms of treatment, but not others?

Session 5. What are the criteria for a 'good' service? The practice members were given the following question to consider:

'You have 2 months to go before the end of the financial year. You only have £25 000 to spend. You must decide which of the health interventions available to you are worthy of funding to get the best value for money. What criteria will you use to decide which "treatments" are better than others?'

Session 6. Practical session: objective setting.

Session 7. Practical session: option appraisal.

Session 8. Decision making:
- A possible system which could be used to develop an agreed 'value' for different referrals
- Factors essential for operating any system for determining priorities.

Session 9. Decision making:
- Devising important criteria for valuing referrals (see Table 7.1)
- Planning the way ahead after the project.

*Based on an article on this subject (Ayres 1996).

EXAMPLE 4. OFFERING PUBLIC HEALTH ADVICE TO A MULTIFUND
*Dr D. Chase and Dr S. Corlett,
Central London Multifund*

Objectives

The multifund developed from a locality advisory group which operated between 1992 and 1994. It is made up of approximately 40 GPs from 21 practices with 12 different funds, and covers 89 000 patients with a budget of £15 million. The multifund provides the opportunity to share expertise and support and enforce clinically driven decisions to achieve greater value for money. One of the objectives of the multifund was to influence service provision in two areas – dermatology referrals and back pain management, with a public health specialist.

Dermatology review

Process

This speciality was prioritized for review because of the high number of GP referrals. The work undertaken included:

- Interviews with GPs and consultants
- Establishing patient satisfaction issues through focus groups
- Analysis of referral data.

Findings

The results revealed the need for:

- Easy and quick access to outpatients
- More feedback from consultants

and identified that:

- 13 dermatology departments received referrals during the preparatory year. The data was poor and mainly of use for accounting purposes rather than assessment of need
- GP referrals were made according to geographical proximity, personal experience and anecdotal experience rather than systematic evaluation of outcomes
- Proactive dermatology departments could demonstrate models of good practice relating to a specialist nurse role, day care and patient support
- Patients' comments can assist the development of quality standards but the value depends on investment of time, expertise and adequate resources
- Two practices in the multifund had dermatology expertise which could provide minor dermatology surgery services.

Impact

The actions listed below ensued:

1. Contracts were focused on three main providers
2. Quality specifications were introduced within the contracts
3. A GP minor cryotherapy service was opened to all practices.

Back pain management

Process

Back pain was identified as a problem because of a 6 month wait for outpatient assessment. Information on who was attending as an outpatient could not be obtained, so it was decided to look at the issue from the perspective of the problems that GPs face when caring for patients with back problems.

- Nine scenarios were devised, ranging from a 22-year-old man with acute pain to a 75-year-old woman with chronic pain
- These scenarios were sent to GPs to ask how they would manage each case
- These scenarios were also sent to consultants in orthopaedics and rheumatology, physiotherapists, and practitioners in acupuncture and osteopathy to ask how GPs should manage the cases
- Opinions were discussed at a multidisciplinary meeting, where those present contributed as clinicians rather than as providers
- Guidelines were drawn up at the meeting
- National guidelines issued by the Clinical Standards Advisory Group were incorporated
- Guidelines were agreed by the GPs
- Guidelines were produced as laminated A4 sheets.

Impact

1. Arrangements for audit of use of guidelines were agreed
2. Specifications were drawn up with orthopaedic surgeons for the back pain clinic, including referrals, being based on guidelines for a multidisciplinary clinic with rapid access
3. Interest in tendering was expressed by five local providers.

Overall impact

Various conclusions were drawn from the experience of assessing these services:

1. Available information is not adequate for making commissioning decisions. A long-term collaborative approach between GPs, the health authority and providers is likely to be more effective than confrontation based on minimal evidence or a single issue.

2. GPs initially wanted organizational solutions to problems, such as consultant outreach clinics or alternative providers. Subsequently it was recognized that their strengths lie in understanding and assessing the clinical aspects of commissioning, and that real improvements in services could be achieved by addressing the wider clinical issues in both primary and secondary care.

3. Understanding the importance of the clinical aspects of contracts led to the recognition that unlimited choice of provider may limit quality. There is merit in working closely with a small number of providers to achieve clinical and other quality standards.

4. Public health skills did usefully contribute to the evaluation and audit of service provision. GPs welcomed access to practical public health skills and would employ public health specialists if resources were available.

5. GPs saw the health authority agenda as rigid and hard to influence. It remains difficult to encourage GPs to link into strategy development, but concentrating on speciality specific review helped to widen GPs' concepts of how service provision can be influenced.

EXAMPLE 5. APPROPRIATE PURCHASING THROUGH NEEDS ASSESSMENT
Dr D. Colin Thome, Castlefields Health Centre, Runcorn, Cheshire

Objectives

In a primary care-led NHS, comprehensive needs assessment should be undertaken at the practice population level, in order to set appropriate priorities and meet them within existing resources. Essentially, this practice sees health needs assessment as the means of creating a picture, which can set the direction for both primary and secondary care services.

The Castlefields practice needs assessment initiative was based on three aspects, as described below.

Use of information technology

Process

General practice is a highly computerized part of the health service, and yet the investment has produced limited information. The Castlefields Health Centre has adopted a paperless system, so that all clinical contacts are entered into computer records using the Read morbidity codes. The database is therefore the product of some 40 000 contacts per year arising from the 12 000 practice population. Community nurses and the social care manager input into the database, as well as practice employed staff.

Impact

1. The database was utilized for future planning at the practice level, and, as comparative data emerge from other practices, can be aggregated for health authority use.

2. Clinical and organizational audit of practice activity can be simplified by use of the database, and can be used to challenge ineffective and inappropriate care whether in primary or secondary care, often releasing money which can be used for wider health needs. As an example, audit of radiography referrals using the Royal College of Radiologists' guidelines resulted in referrals falling by some 30%, allowing for development of other services such as community nursing.

Obtaining community feedback

Process

This was undertaken in three ways: regular meetings with local councillors, a health forum formed from local residents, and a survey of patient opinions. Councillors brought a knowledge of the community and expertise in representing the community's views. The health forum provided an opportunity to exchange views on health and health related matters, and a safe place to make criticisms and explore complaints. Proposals for contract changes were also discussed with the forum. The survey covered 8% of the practice population, asking for views on appointments, home visits, receptionists, disabled access, consultations and the overall view of the service.

Impact

The responses to the survey formed the basis for the development of the patients charter for the practice.

The public health role

Process

This was developed through a 2 year project undertaken by a public health nurse, using various techniques including appraisal of small-area census information, and interviewing of key people in the community.

Findings

The work identified substantial causes of mortality such as coronary heart disease and cancer. Wider health needs were also identified such as environmental quality (housing, lighting, etc.), prevention of accidents, the need for parenting skills, and the health needs of young people.

Impact

1. The work of the primary health care team was focused on a systematic approach to prevention, care, treatment and rehabilitation of the major causes of death.

2. Local community initiatives to address the wider health needs included a teenage health project and work with a local housing association.

Conclusions

The Castlefields experience shows that needs assessment can be undertaken by the primary care team, but it must be an essential part of caring for people and enhancing the health of communities, not a bureaucratic process done because it is the current fashion. It has been the key building block enabling the practice to develop care in response to needs and shift resources from secondary to primary care, thus facilitating the development of community services.

EXAMPLE 6. NEEDS ASSESSMENT AND TOTAL PURCHASING
Bromsgrove GP Total Purchasing Project, Bromsgrove, Worcestershire

Objectives

The objectives were to conduct needs assessment as part of a broad public health physician's contribution to a GP total purchasing project (see Box 7.4).

Process

Bromsgrove is a small, well-circumscribed town just south of Birmingham. There are four fundholding practices in the town, providing care to about 40 000 patients. The total purchasing project started in April 1994.

The opportunities for achieving change are much greater with total purchasing than with fundholding or health authority purchasing, because the GPs have flexi-bility to influence the whole range of primary and secondary care services directly. This is reflected in the range of issues covered by formal population-based needs assessment or service evaluation (Table 7.2).

The involvement of public health physicians in the Bromsgrove GP Total Purchasing Project has been extensive, with an experienced senior registrar assigned to the project for a nominal 2 days per week, although actually committing much more time than this. However, part of this commitment is actually undertaking comparisons with the wider district populations, and therefore contributing to the understanding of need and service effectiveness at the macro level. Nevertheless, it is evident from our experience that primary care total purchasing will not result in a reduced role for the public health function. Indeed, the need for practice-based data analysis and regular communications with the practices suggests that the time commitment in this example of one of whole time equivalent practitioner per 100 000 population is the minimum requirement, although unlikely to be feasible given the current pressures on the management costs of health authorities.

Box 7.4 Objectives – public health roles in total purchasing in Bromsgrove

1. Provision of practical public health skills to the project:
   - Provide skills, time and knowledge
   - Introduce public health values and attitudes to complement general practice values
   - Encourage the development of analysis and evaluation skills in the practice
   - Undertake analysis of comparative data between project population and district population.
2. Relating total purchasing to strategy and policy:
   - Ensuring the district population is not disadvantaged by the actions of the total purchasers
   - Challenging proposed changes on grounds of clinical and cost-effectiveness
   - Negotiating agreements in situations of clinical and professional conflict
   - Prioritizing dedicated public health time to total purchasing.

Table 7.2 Health needs assessment and service evaluations

Assessment area	Investigations and impact
Health of the Nation priorities	
Coronary heart disease	Population needs assessment and development of prevention strategy
Cerebrovascular disease	Population needs assessment, management protocols for care on GP ward, improvements in rehabilitation services
Mental illness	Population needs assessment, contribution to district review and strategy development
Community services	
Family planning	Demand, access and quality requirements Extended range of GP family planning clinics
Minor injury service	Review of activity of nurse run service Evaluation of outcomes of GP involvement
Leg ulcer care	Assessment of need and modern treatments Establishment of specialist clinic and monitoring of cure rates
Respite care	Assessment of need and contract with nursing homes for care provision
GP-managed beds in the community	Effect of proactive management on length of stay in hospital and outcomes
Acute services	
Emergency medical admissions	Year-on-year activity comparisons, access rates by practice, peer review of admission behaviour, primary care-driven early discharge, extended use of low-technology facilities, e.g. nursing homes and community beds
Antenatal care	Review of antenatal visit protocols, transfer of some hospital clinic visits to midwives in GP surgery

Impact (Table 7.2)

1. There was mutual learning of general practice and public health values and skills.

2. Improvements were made in existing services, e.g. stroke and GP family planning clinics.

3. New services were begun, e.g. leg ulcer clinics and a new respite care contract.

4. Primary care controlled the interface with the secondary sector, promoting earlier discharges to low-technology beds, and some antenatal care transferred to primary care.

IMPLICATIONS AND LESSONS LEARNT

The examples in this chapter demonstrate a range of approaches and attitudes to achieving improved health care through primary care purchasing.

How realistic can we be in expecting needs assessment to be the driving force in GP purchasing, can we reduce the barriers which may influence this, and what role does needs assessment take in fundholder purchasing? For most GPs starting out in fundholding, initial plans focus on the needs of individual patients and improved access to services which have traditionally been available. As experience grows and resources come under increasing pressure, interest begins to turn to the practice population as a whole, with its range of needs and the consequences of deciding priorities. For most GPs, needs assessment comes secondary to the practicalities of negotiating a budget and agreeing contracts. This must be accepted if needs assessment is to be encouraged as a longer-term strategy. Needs assessment can seem formal and remote, based on population estimates, which, while meaningful to public health physicians who work with such data on a daily basis, may seem distant to the GP and the patient in front of him. Recognizing the difference in culture and values, and accepting these differences as complementary rather than conflicting, is an important step towards incorporating needs assessment into practice plans.

GP fundholding is undertaken within an accountability framework set out in EL (95) 54, which 'deals primarily with GP fundholders' management accountability and their accountability to patients and the public. It also sets out existing arrangements for clinical, professional and financial accountability.' The emphasis in this guidance is on 'the principle of GPs using their knowledge and judgement to best meet patients' needs.' It talks about GP fundholders working in partnership with health authorities, primarily health care teams and local NHS trusts, to develop and implement locally agreed health and service strategies. It describes the role of the annual practice plan in setting out how the practice intends to use its fund and the practice's contribution to targets and priorities. It does not step back to the stage of needs assessment at the practice level in order to define priorities for both primary and secondary care. Needs assessment will become a significant feature only if GPs themselves, or local PHPs, act as product champions and demonstrate in a practical way how the techniques can contribute to effective purchasing.

NEEDS ASSESSMENT AND INFORMATION

Clearly, accurate needs assessment needs accurate data, which can be interpreted and analysed in order to form the basis for decisions on resource use. This is evident from all the examples described, with attempts to use a wide range of data sources. A common problem running through the examples is the inadequacy of most of the databases to support primary care needs assessments. Fundholding information technology systems are more suitable for paying invoices from providers than identifying the need which led to the episode of care (see Ch. 13). Population databases and national data such as the census are normally compiled on a geographical basis, and can therefore only give broad indicators according to the proportion of the practice population residing within a defined small area (see Ch. 4).

Increasingly, it will become evident that the 'top down' epidemiological estimate approach to needs assessment must be replaced by actual assessment of need at practice level, and that primary care information technology systems must support this, particularly with clinically relevant information on activity and analysis of patient dependency. Effective resource use depends on a high level of detail on need, enabling the GP purchaser to estimate such things as the number of hospital or community attendances for each patient, and the staff requirements in terms of skill mix. Already it is evident that the imaginative use of existing systems can achieve much, and the increasing interest of fundholders in assessing needs should provide the stimulus for developing systems to support this function.

INVOLVING SERVICE USERS AND PROVIDERS

As the emphasis of needs assessment moves to practice level, the involvement of service users and carers in surveys and focus groups will extend. Formal surveys of health problems and experience of service use can add to the knowledge acquired on an anecdotal basis, and can provide more objective evidence on which to base decisions, especially where shifts of work between providers is involved. Some of the examples illustrate the longer-term benefits to be achieved by working with providers to make clinical services more effective and appropriate rather than simply focusing on organizational arrangements, or transferring the work and leaving other purchasers to suffer the consequences.

With increased understanding of needs comes increased interest in effectively meeting need, with quality of clinical care becoming a key issue. The cycle of needs assessment includes a review of current research and development issues and current approaches to management, so it is hardly surprising that astute purchasers start to define the standards of clinical care required for their investment. In geographical areas where a large choice of providers can be accessed, this is likely to lead to a 'preferred provider' approach which can be compared with the US model of managed care organizations.

THE ROLE OF THE HEALTH AUTHORITY

With the establishment of the new health authorities in April 1996 bringing together responsibility for primary care provision and undertaking or overseeing secondary care purchasing, it is necessary to move from a more directive to a more facilitative style of management. The role defined in EL (94) 79, *Developing NHS Purchasing and GP Fundholding*, was that of strategy, monitoring and support, with a strong partnership between health authorities and GPs. It is clear from some of the examples described that skills commonly found in health authorities, particularly information analysis and public health, can usefully be shared with GPs as they move forward the primary care-led NHS agenda. The cultural shift from a 'top down' needs assessment defining a 'top down' strategy to that of practice based needs assessments aggregating to form a strategic overview is significant, and will not be achieved without mutual recognition of the skills and values of each part of the organization.

THE OPPORTUNITIES OF FUNDHOLDING

Fundholding offers a flexible approach to contracting and resource use which has achieved rapid changes in the NHS. The control of patients and their care has moved away from secondary care, as GPs increasingly define their expectation of the consultant and his intervention in the patient care programme. In the early years of fundholding, with limited procedures within the fund, this shift was confined to relatively well-circumscribed aspects of care. Now, with fundholding extending through standard and community funds to total purchasing, the entire range of services is coming under scrutiny. GPs are increasingly looking for 'added value' from the services they purchase, a demonstration that some benefit can be achieved beyond that which they can provide themselves. With budgets as real money, reducing access to secondary care can result in savings which can be invested to achieve real extensions in the care available within the practice. It is incumbent on GPs to ensure that the services they provide themselves are kept under the same active scrutiny as those which they purchase from traditional providers.

CONCLUSIONS

This chapter has illustrated a number of practical ways in which practices are using more or less sophisticated approaches to needs assessment in order to help provide and purchase the best possible services for their patients. The science and art of needs assessment will continue to develop, and it is essential that this takes account of the practical use to which the techniques will be put. Primary care-led purchasing will lead the NHS into the next millennium, regardless of whether the precise mechanism is fundholding or some alternative key influence on resource use. Needs assessment must be the essential building block from which the cycle of purchasing starts, and this will only happen with positive support and a pragmatic approach to the task.

REFERENCES

Ayres P J 1996 Rationing health care: views from general practice. Social Science and Medicine (in press)
Hewett G, Mein G, Brown E, Evans T, Milner A 1994 Into informed purchasing: 1. District nursing. Commissioning services for patients' needs: a needs assessment study in primary care. Paxton Green Group Practice, London.

ACKNOWLEDGEMENT

Particular thanks are due to Dr Paul Watson, Director of Acute Services, Cambridge and Huntingdon Health Authority, for research provided in this chapter.

8

Locality needs assessment

Jane Hopton   George Leahy

INTRODUCTION

At the core of locality health needs assessment are two major issues. First, locality health needs assessment must address the issue of what localities are in terms of their function and structure, not just as a geographic or administrative base. Second, there is the uncertainty about the relationship between health needs assessment and commissioning (Salter 1993). This uncertainty is not unique to locality-based health needs assessment, but the diversity of locality commissioning models, the political debate about this approach to commissioning, and the fact that developments are continuing apace brings it in to focus.

In this context of organizational change and uncertainty, the relationship between health needs assessment and the commissioning process is at best unclear – some might say non-existent. Those involved in the development of locality commissioning frameworks and structures often see health needs as esoteric, irrelevant and incomprehensible. Those involved in locality health needs assessment are frequently frustrated by their inability to inform decision making, and bring about change and development.

The challenge for locality health needs assessment is to make explicit, and understand the links between, the purpose, principles and process of health needs assessment and to seek to integrate them in the commissioning process.

This chapter has been made possible by surveying practice in the field. But first we must consider 'what is a locality?'

LOCALITIES: MORE THAN AN ISSUE OF GEOGRAPHY AND ADMINISTRATION

In a general analysis of the concept of space in British health policy, Moon (1990) identified three primary functions, and these present a useful starting point to consider the development of locality commissioning structures and needs assessment. Firstly, geographical areas are defined for formal or administrative purposes, for example for resource allocation and management. Geographical areas also function as a focus for localism, that is, as a way of focusing on people's needs and views, as a focus for interprofessional work.

Moon (1990) also provides a political analysis of these functions. Gerrymandering is a familiar acknowledgement of the link between geographical areas and political priorities. The idea that planning should be more locally sensitive has been embraced by both right and left. On the right, the move to more local structures offers a devolution or abnegation of state responsibility and accountability, with the promotion of an ideology of self-reliance. This interpretation can easily lead to avoidance of social and structural issues; self-help may be instrumental to cost cutting. For the left, more local structures offer local democracy and empowerment. Taken together, the fine line between these political approaches highlights the importance of looking closely for the different interpretations and implications of similar rhetoric about localities (Plampling & Delamothe 1991).

The impact of national policy on current concepts of locality

Since the 1990 National Health Service (NHS) reforms a wide range of commissioning models have developed. Two aspects of the reforms have substantially influenced locality developments – the primary care-led NHS and consumerism. The move towards a primary care-led NHS, with general practice fundholding (GPFH) at the core of this shift, has had two strands of influence on commissioning models. One effect was to encourage local development of commissioning models as alternatives to fundholding (Gaffy & Williams 1994, Wainwright 1996). These models have been referred to collectively under the umbrella term 'locality' models. In broad terms the development of these models represented an attempt to build on concepts of equity, strategy and cooperation rather than competition as a basis for planning and development. The difference between 'locality' and fundholding models of commissioning has recently become somewhat obscured: GPFHs have cooperated with each other to achieve economies of scale and develop strategies for financial risk management (Fettes 1994), and many locality commissioning organizations are seeking to manage funds directly (Wainwright 1996). The implications of the different political frameworks of the models have not yet been systematically explored. However, one implication appears to be the difference in visibility of the commissioning process, including health needs assessment. By attempting to work cooperatively and strategically, locality commissioning groups inevitably increase their visibility and until recently have been unprotected, by working outwith national policy.

The second effect of the reforms has been to place general practitioners (GPs) at the core of the commissioning process, and to pressure locality models to be general practice led (Morley 1993, National Association of Commissioning Groups 1995). This not only influences the corporate structure of locality commissioning but encourages the localities to be geographically as well as conceptually based on general practices. It has implications for localities as a focus for interprofessional work, raising questions about the roles, input and accountability of other primary health care, public health and social welfare professionals (Young & Haynes 1993, Canning 1994), especially in the development of joint planning for community care.

Consumerism has been a key theme in the introduction of market principles and localities are also seen as areas for public consultation. Locality developments on this theme have been somewhat overwhelmed and obscured by developments in commissioning which have primarily focused on health professionals as proxy reporters of consumer views and secondarily focused on health professionals as researchers or collectors of consumer views. Locality commissioning structures which directly involve local people are at present relatively rare (Ham 1992).

The impact of local politics on concepts of locality

Against this backdrop, a diversity of commissioning structures and processes are being implemented locally. How structures have been developed and implemented has received little systematic scrutiny. Nevertheless, discussions with contributors to this chapter about their health needs assessment work were bound-up with descriptions of the local structures and how these structures had developed. One commissioning agency defined its localities primarily to be coterminous with local authority boundaries, with the exception of two localities where boundaries were adjusted to accommodate GPs who identified more clearly with GPs in a different local authority area than their own. Another commissioning agency positively chose to work with geographic and issue-based groups of GPs. Some 'localities' were based on natural geographic areas (for example, general practices based within the same town), whereas in order to develop the commissioning input of inner-city general practices, it was recognized that small practices with large ethnic minority populations formed a more natural group than practices grouped arbitrarily by geography. The boundaries of a third locality, working with a community development model, were adjusted in order to meet the qualifying criteria for an Urban Aid Grant.

In short, concepts and interpretations of locality are not straightforward and can embrace a wide range of structural interests and ideologies. In practice, localities have different corporate structures reflecting their different functions, accountability, remits, resources and political origins (Ham 1992, Meethan & Thompson 1993). At a concrete level, they cover different sizes of populations and geographic area. For example, in an early review of locality structures, Ham (1992) described localities corresponding to natural communities such as small towns or villages of between 8000 and 20 000 people, ranging to those corresponding to district and borough council areas of 100 000 people. These aspects of localities are continually evolving and, more importantly, all have implications for the process and methods and relevance of health needs assessment.

TOWARDS INTEGRATION: A FRAMEWORK FOR ASSESSING LOCALITY HEALTH NEEDS ASSESSMENTS

This section describes an analytical framework for assessing locality health needs assessments (Box 8.1). The framework is heuristic, being devised partly on the basis of theory and partly on the basis of the health needs assessment work reviewed. For this reason, different case studies illustrate different aspects of the framework, and we selectively refer to case studies which are described in more detail in a separate section below. The purpose of the framework is to encourage critical reflection on the links between health needs assessments and locality commissioning structures and functions, and the processes of decision making and strategy development at locality level.

Box 8.1 A framework for assessing locality health needs assessments

Purpose	● Strategic ● Operational
Principles	● Concepts of needs ● Philosophy of methods/approach

Process	● Stages of health needs assessment:
	  – Needs identification
	  – Option generation
	  – Option appraisal
	  – Prioritization of options
	  – Implementation and evaluation
	  – Review locality strategy
	● Data and methods
	● Organization
	● Pitfalls

The purpose of health needs assessment

In broad terms it is possible to distinguish between health needs assessments which are strategic and those which are operational. By strategic we mean those which are undertaken to provide a resource or to inform broad-based medium-term plans for development. Locality or practice profiles such as those undertaken by Barking and Havering, Bexley and Greenwich, Leicestershire and Lothian exemplify this approach (Box 8.2). Profiles which focus on routine data can be supplemented by other data to produce 'community profiles' (see Ch. 11). In contrast, operational needs assessments are those undertaken to inform development in areas already identified as being of strategic importance, or core business. These may be geographical areas, e.g. areas of social deprivation (The West Central Halifax Project), or groups within the population, e.g. the elderly (The Salford Elders Project), or where specific decisions have to be made, e.g. siting new services (The Wirral Oncology Project).

Consideration clearly has to be given to the relationship between these approaches. Operational needs assessments are, by definition, more narrowly focused and more closely linked with change and resources. Both the West Central Halifax and Salford operational needs assessment projects were carried out in response to the availability of targeted resources. Prioritization of these needs assessments may or may not have reflected locality priorities identified by broader exploratory profiles of need.

Box 8.2 Barking and Havering: health and social profiles of localities

Size of locality	Approximately 55 000 people
Objective	To inform primary and community health teams of the main features of the social structure of the locality and of associated health problems
Process	Analysis of routine data sets by locality profiles
Findings	Census data on age and sex structure, ethnicity, deprivation, tenure and social class, general practice data on health promotion and the following morbidity and mortality data: long-term illness, psychiatric admissions, heart disease, stroke, cancers, suicides and accidents, and infant mortality rates
Impact	Not known, but in as far as they are done without reference to users of data, and that service provision was not included, minimal

---

The principles of health needs assessment

Health needs assessment also incorporates a set of principles or values. Although these are often not made explicit, they are implicit in concepts of needs and in the methods or approach (Hopton & Dlugolecka 1995a) and have important links with the politics of locality planning. There is a great temptation to make reference to 'methods', in order to sidestep the discomforts of conflicting values and interests. However, making values explicit is not only a moral issue, it can also be a practical one since principles and values inevitably form part of the negotiation of decisions or corporate commitment to change (Kitsuse & Spector 1973).

Three differing interpretations of need are of particular relevance, those of comparative need, normative need and corporate need (Bradshaw 1972). Comparative need relates directly to the principle of equity. Comparisons can be made amongst localities which could give indications for resource allocation, or amongst practice populations or smaller areas within localities to give indications for resource redistribution (Hopton & Dlugolecka 1995b).

Normative need is that defined by experts, professionals, doctors or policy makers, and identification of unmet need is based on the discrepancy between the desirable and existing standards. It should be recognized that lay people can be experts (Popay & Williams 1994). The definition of 'expert' should always remain contestable. Definitions of normative need often focus on specific subgroups within the populations, although what constitutes a subgroup is diverse and could be people experiencing a particular illness, ethnic minorities or people living within a particular area. Normative need can be characterized by statements such as, 'there should be 600 coronary artery bypass grafts per 100 000 people (British Cardiac Society).

The concept of corporate need is that which recognizes a range of perspectives including professionals and lay people, and may also take into account the interest principles or parameters imposed by the commissioning organization including, for example, availability of resources and wide policy priorities.

Whilst the distinction between these concepts of need is conceptually important, in practice they are closely related to the purpose and process of health needs assessments, and the distinctions may become integrated. For example, comparative approaches to needs identification are of particular value in considering resource redistribution and for strategic needs assessments via comprehensive comparative profiles. Where comparative profiles have indicated areas of unmet need in broad terms, then a normative approach may be required to develop a more detailed understanding of the needs in order to generate options to address these needs (see, for example, The Lothian Five Practice Study described on p. 99).

The principles of a health needs assessment can be described in broad terms, independently of the concepts of need. For example, The West Central Halifax Project used the principles of community development, in broad terms empowering local people to bring about sustainable environmental and social change to address inequalities in health and socioeconomic status. The starting position of the project was to look at how the culture of organizations such as health centres or hospitals clashed with that of local users of those institutions.

The process of health needs assessment

Health needs assessment should be seen as a process integrated with commissioning although it is often misleadingly seen in terms of 'independent' methods. There are some approaches which are frequently referred to as 'methods' such as multimethod, rapid appraisal or participatory appraisal which seem to imply both a set of principles and a process, yet often fail to make either explicit (Milburn et al 1995, Hopton & Dlugolecka 1995a).

This is not to imply that health needs assessment does not depend upon methodological rigour, but the methodological appropriateness and rigour have to be considered in terms of the process as a whole as some methods may be more appropriate at different stages of the process.

Some localities have taken the important step of defining their own process of health needs assessment. For example, the Worth Valley Health Consortium process is illustrated in Box 8.3.

Box 8.3 Worth Valley Health Consortium: needs assessment process

1. Prioritization of areas for needs assessments
2. Consider these priorities in the context of local and national priorities
3. Develop a clear and precise definition of the problem
4. Assess the epidemiology
5. Review existing evidence about standards of practice and solutions to the problem
6. Undertake a service review
7. Incorporate the views of a range of stakeholders including professional and lay perspectives
8. Identify further information and research requirements and develop recommendations for action

---

Stages of health needs assessment

The process of health needs assessment can be considered in the following stages:

1. Needs identification
2. Option generation
3. Option appraisal
4. Prioritization of options
5. Implementation and evaluation
6. Review locality strategy.

This process is related to the purpose of the needs assessments. For example, strategic needs assessments identify typical need rather than assess options to meet need, and as such rarely progress beyond the first stage. Most of the case study material reported here covered only one or two of these stages. Case-finding or screening approaches can be used to identify unmet need (see Ch. 9). One example of this is the recording of preventative aspects of care in a network of GP practices in east London (Table 8.1), which showed a low uptake of breast screening by ethnic minorities. This led to discussions in the local community and a GP being commissioned to investigate and advise on service delivery strategy and appointment of ethnic community advocates, who dramatically improved uptake.

It is also important to note that there is nothing inevitable about this process. Identification of need does not automatically lead to option generation. For example, the Lothian survey carried out in five general practices clearly identified areas of relative unmet need, yet multidisciplinary discussion groups held in each practice identified very few options for addressing these areas of need, and when these were identified they were expressed in very broad terms. Both The Lothian Five Practice Project and The West Central Halifax Project noted the gulf between knowing that something needs to be done and suggesting what could be done, the familiar difficulty of imagining how things could be different without experience (Porter & MacIntyre 1994) that exists for both lay people and professionals.

Two examples of needs assessments which were undertaken within what could be broadly described as a developmental approach (The West Central Halifax Project and The Salford Elders Project) covered these stages in a more explicit way and used different methods appropriate to the different stages of the process.

In the Salford project, once needs had been identified using routine epidemiological data and a social survey, these were discussed in a multidisciplinary setting to generate all possible options and to agree the content and importance of criteria for option appraisal (Box 8.4). The criteria made explicit both the principles, such as equity or economic viability, as well as the expertise of stakeholders, such as the importance given to the options by service users. A second survey of the relevant population was carried out to allow local people to appraise the options.

Data and methods for health needs assessment

Given the diversity in size of areas and populations of localities, let alone their structures and functions, there is

---

Box 8.4 The Salford Elders Project: option appraisal criteria

- Should be consistent with the views of older people
- Consistent with local workers' views
- Give value for money
- Be feasible
- Consistent with the priorities of relevant organizations
- Should promote equity
- Be consistent with GPs' priorities
- Were likely to be effective

---

no 'off the peg' best locality approach. The key methodological issues are largely created by the problems of defining localities in terms of conflicting functions (resource allocation, interprofessional working and assessing the needs of local populations) and conflicts of interests (lay versus professional views) (Bullen et al 1996; Box 8.5).

Box 8.5 Key methodological issues in locality needs assessments

1. Reliability
2. Coterminosity
3. Aggregation
4. People versus place
5. Relevance of different methods at different stages of the process

---

Reliability. Issues of reliability of different data sources used at different area levels are addressed elsewhere (see Chs 2 and 6). However, it is worth noting here that consideration should be given to the reliability of data for small areas, particularly for rare conditions or events. If data cannot be sufficiently reliable, should they be collected for a larger area, or not be collected at all?

Coterminosity. The issue of coterminous boundaries and populations comes to the fore in the context of localities, particularly when localities are defined in terms of general practice populations. General practice populations are typically diffuse and do not correspond to postcode sector, enumeration districts or wards. For example, it is possible that two general practices sharing a catchment area and a geographic population could have practice populations that are very different in terms of age, sex and socioeconomic status. Integrating or comparing individual data held by practices, health services, local authorities and the census requires care. General practice

---

Table 8.1 Needs assessment of acceptability of screening tests to different cultures. Percentage differences in recording aspects of preventative care in a network of GP practices in east London (The Healthy Eastenders Project)

	White (n = 187)	Black (n = 85)	Bangladeshi (n = 107)	Chinese/Vietnamese (n = 102)
Cervical smear (%)	88	82	86	82
Breast radiography (%)	46	22	17	20

population profiles based on census data can be produced via postcodes of individual patients, as they are for allocation of the deprivation allowance. Geographical information systems make this approach more feasible, but this is not straightforward (Twigg 1990).

This issue of coterminosity in the analysis of quantitative data has its counterpart in terms of the meaningfulness of qualitative data at locality, sublocality or practice level. Many of the needs assessments reviewed incorporate qualitative data collected from interviews with health professionals and sometimes with lay people as experts, on the needs of a population. Few needs assessments have reflected on the meaningfulness of asking them to do so. For example, whilst lay people may be important informants of the health needs of themselves and their own immediate 'natural' communities, could lay people meaningfully comment on the needs of a general practice population or a locality? At a similar, though perhaps less obvious, level, to what extent can professionals be asked meaningfully about the needs of practice or locality populations if these do not correspond to the populations with which they work and are familiar?

Aggregation. The issue of aggregation has to be considered both in terms of data and in terms of strategy development.

In terms of data there are known hazards in making assumptions that data and interpretations of data aggregated at one level apply to other lower levels. The dangers of ecological fallacy, that is, that false assumptions are made about individuals, have been well documented. This is a particular problem for large localities and raises the question of 'how local is local?' and may need to be divided into smaller sublocality areas or practice populations for planning, but the issue is also relevant at sublocality or practice level as critics of the allocation of the deprivation allowance have already highlighted (Sheldon et al 1991). Pockets of deprivation and need are easily missed.

Thought also needs to be given to whether needs assessments or strategies developed in sublocalities or general practices can be meaningfully aggregated to the locality strategy. For example, work in Bradford surveyed in detail the views of practices on service provision and areas for development. The content of the responses of each practice was summed to produce a locality profile in terms of the frequency with which issues were raised. It may be that a different sampling strategy, for example sampling a range of professionals within the locality rather than sampling practices, would have produced a different profile.

People versus place. Much of the data that are used in health needs assessment is information about individuals which is aggregated to different levels. Moreover, aggregated data are frequently used as ways of describing areas. Work on the allocation of resources typically uses

formulas based on aggregated data on individuals to describe areas in terms of degree of deprivation. The development of social marketing has brought a range of sophisticated approaches to classifying areas in terms of their resident population. The 'Super Profile' classification used in the Wirral exemplifies this approach (Table 8.2).

Whilst these classifications are used to examine the links between environment and health, in essence all these approaches are based on individuals rather than focusing on place as a determinant of health (MacIntyre et al 1993). Moreover, they can overlook the fact that data can mean different things in different places. For example, car ownership has a different meaning in rural settings. Similarly amongst the needs assessments reviewed, some locality profiles were based solely on social or clinical epidemiological data about individuals whereas others acknowledged the importance of place.

The relevance of different methods at different stages of the process. The sections above have begun to explore some of the possibilities for using methods at different stages of the health needs assessment process. In the stage of assessing current services, observational studies, although very time-consuming, allow the assessor to see what is actually happening (see Ch. 5). Qualitative methods of assessing individual user's perceptions of health care needs are summarized in Table 8.3.

The work in Salford highlighted the potential of multidisciplinary discussion groups for generating options and criteria at the option appraisal stage. The process defined by the Worth Valley draws attention to the potential for systematic literature reviews to be incorporated into the process and the value of doing it before the service review in order to inform the review questions.

By describing in detail the process of health needs assessment it is possible to identify where different values or principles come into play and how different methods have the potential to incorporate these values. For example, a range of criteria can be used to appraise options including normative criteria based on the

Table 8.2 'Super Profile' lifestyle categories – original and amended descriptive names

Original name	Amended name (used in Wirral[a])
Affluent achievers	Affluent professionals
Thriving greys	Better-off older people
Settled suburbans	Settled suburbia
Nest builders	Better-off young families
Urban venturers	Younger/mobile
Country life	Rural communities
Senior citizens	Lower income older people
Producers	Blue collar workers
Hard-pressed families	Lower income households
Have nots	Lowest income households

[a] For use in planning health care services it was considered that slightly different descriptive names would be more appropriate than those used originally.

Table 8.3 Qualitative methods of surveying expressed needs

In-depth interviews	Focus groups	Nominal group technique
Time-consuming Interviewer needs training Flexible Good for gathering data on personal and private experience	Exploratory Some groups do not work Experienced facilitator needed Good for finding range of stake-holder views and stimulating responses at an early stage Can access cultural or shared knowledge	Less threatening, but less rich discussion than instructed focus groups Good at balancing views of consumers and various professionals

opinion of experts, economic criteria, criteria based on principles of equity and empowerment. Consensus methods could be used to agree upon criteria, as was the case in the Salford project.

This project tailored its questionnaires to enable respondents to reach a consensus. It is crucially important that managers and doctors alike take proper advice in designing and piloting any questionnaire, if its results are to have any validity or reliability. A brief guide to the key criteria can be found in Table 2.3.

Nominal group technique is particularly suited to prevent bias from vocal professionals dominating discussions (see Box 8.6).

It is possible to use forms of systematic appraisals, which make direct reference to a particular policy approach. Marginal analysis, an economic approach, has found application in a broader health needs assessment framework, and represents a form of incrementalism (Lindblom 1959, Cohen 1994). Whatever combination of techniques is used, the importance of using proven methods and only varying them after careful consideration is reiterated (see Ch. 2) (Milburn et al 1995).

Organization

Making the point that health needs assessment requires organization may seem somewhat trivial, but is of new relevance in the context of the development of locality structures, general practice or patch based needs assessments. Although consideration is already being given to the role of public health, particularly where locality structures have developed primarily as a means of incorporating GPs into the commissioning process, less attention has been given to the organization required at general practice or sublocality levels where a range of health professionals could be gathering and interpreting data and information on health needs. More often, their views are being researched as part of the health needs assessment process. The London Project, led from general practice and described in more detail below (see the case studies), developed the potential for interprofessional collaboration in health needs assessment, across sectors of the primary care team, and explored the importance of organizational factors. More recently, a project led from a health agency has emphasized the crucial need for integrated organization across profession and management (The East Kent Locality Commissioning Project (Box 8.7)).

Pitfalls

The important challenge is to identify potential pitfalls at all stages of the health needs assessment process in advance. One of the major pitfalls is to find the resources to meet needs once they have been assessed. The West Central Halifax Project identified short-termism as a potential problem of grant or ad hoc funding, and sought from the outset to consider the sustainability of developments made by considering what the project termed 'exit strategies' to ensure that developments would continue once the project structure was removed.

Box 8.6 Process of nominal group technique

- Choose homogeneous groups (e.g. patients, GPs, consultants, nurses)
- Select 4–8 participants and leaders per group
- Agree on an area/topic for exploration
- Leaders brief groups on technique and task
- Generation phase:
  - individuals silently generate ideas on paper
  - contributions summarized on flipchart
- Discussion phase – group-related ideas
- Scoring phase:
  - group ranking of importance of items and discussion of top 10
  - private individual ranking to produce core data

Box 8.7 East Kent Locality Commissioning Project

Process
In five pilot sites, teams comprising a facilitator, GP, social services manager, locality nurse manager, therapist representative and community health council member were formed. Their qualitative assessments were by questionnaire and interview.

Impact
This project did not identify any issues unknown to the health agency, but four teams wished to address specific areas further in their sites – GP-based physiotherapy, community rehabilitation, training foot care assistants and under five needs assessment. This corporate needs assessment succeeded in engaging general practice in commissioning and improving working relationships, but failed to establish specific aspects of commissioning relevant to the population of localities. The reasons appeared to be unrealistic objectives, insufficient data, appropriate public health expertise not sought early enough, lack of health authority strategy and perceived lack of influence of the project on the authority.

CASE STUDIES

Examples of strategic needs assessment using comparative profiling

Many of the examples of needs assessments reviewed fell into this category, consisting of profiles of localities compared with the region as a whole or comparing smaller areas within a locality, with the locality as a whole, or comparing data from different general practices. A range of data and information sources were incorporated in the profiles, although data and information used were predominantly those which were routinely available. Some of the profiles were focused on specific issues or priorities, in other cases the approach seemed to be to give as comprehensive a profile as possible from available data.

Comparative profiles using routinely available data

Bexley and Greenwich Health: comparative profiles of the seven localities.

Size. Localities are based on populations of around 55 000 and are based on general practices. Localities are further subdivided according to main population centres or wards, and differences between these smaller areas and the locality as a whole are described.

Objective. The locality profiles are seen as an information base or resource which could be used to develop strategy, but are distinct from a strategically commissioned needs assessment.

Process. Analysis of routine data sets and health service activity data.

Finding. The profiles integrate available data about the population (sociodemographic information, routinely available morbidity and mortality data), data about existing services and, where possible, data on service utilization. Detailed descriptions of existing primary care and community services are given, along with an overview of voluntary and social services. Data on service use include prescribing, hospitalization rates, immunization and screening uptake rates and available data on community service activity. The profiles also look at services available for specific population groups: services for people with learning disabilities, mental health problems, alcohol and drug abuse problems and for Black and ethnic minority groups.

Impact. By incorporating data on service provision and use the profiles go beyond looking at the characteristics of people to incorporate information about place, and in turn allow profile summaries to make strategic suggestions for service developments. For example, one ward within a locality had the greatest proportions of older people and highest rates of long-term illness, suggesting that programmes for chronic disease management could be a priority area. A different ward had a high propor-

tion of lone pensioners, and 40% of pensioners' homes in the same area lacked basic amenities, drawing attention to potential problems for hospital discharge planning and community care.

Leicestershire Health: locality gazettes.

Size. Currently there are 14 localities, although consideration is being given to reducing the numbers.

Objective. The primary purpose was to encourage exchange of information amongst practices with a view to developing a strategic approach to local clinical guidelines.

Process. Production of gazettes which are sent to general practices. Data from one practice is compared with the other practices in Leicestershire. The data from the gazettes have been aggregated to the localities although the primary audience for the gazettes is the practice and secondarily the health commission.

Findings. Gazettes produced so far have been based on available data tackling the following issues: diabetes, minor surgery, peptic ulcer disease, smoking, hip and cataract procedures, prescribing analysis and cost tables (PACT) data on prescribing of anti-inflammatory drugs, women and child health including childhood accidents and asthma, availability of female health professionals, hysterectomy and sterilization rates and provision of nursing services.

Impact. The locality gazettes have begun to stimulate debate. For example, one gazette highlighted inequities in practice nurse allocation, while another showed the variation in admission rate due to avoidable complications in diabetes. This could be a useful measure of effective shared care in the community. The primary focus is on practice development, and the usefulness of the approach is seen to depend very much on the extent to which the gazettes provoke constructive discussion within practices. Leicestershire health professionals have taken the important step of beginning an evaluation of their approach in terms of both the format and the nature of the information distributed.

Population surveys and comparative profiling

All the above approaches have been based on routinely available data. As a direct consequence of being routinely available much of the data on morbidity is dependent upon service availability and use. Similarly existing data on service use are difficult to interpret unless data on community morbidity are also available to give an indication of whether patterns of availability and use of services are appropriate, or whether there are areas of unmet need. Population surveys offer the opportunity to overcome the drawbacks of routinely available data. They also offer the opportunity of incorporating users' perceptions of health and illness and their views on service provision and priorities for development overcoming a further omission from the comparative approaches reviewed above.

In Lothian, two surveys have been carried out. The first was a large stratified random sample survey of the population of Lothian as a whole, which has allowed comparison by locality. The second survey is described below (Box 8.8).

Both principal survey researchers made substantial efforts to clarify the purpose of the survey and consulted widely with relevant health care professionals about the content of the survey instrument in the hope that this would increase the relevance and likelihood of the work having a practical impact. With one or two notable exceptions, it proved very difficult to obtain the input of practitioners and planners. Even open questions about what information would be interesting or useful to them brought little response. This suggests that although practitioners and policy makers can easily spot information that is not relevant or useful, they are perhaps less able to identify their information needs strategically. Again this makes the point that despite the power of the method, and surveys are a very powerful and flexible method, translating health needs assessments into relevant implications and action depends upon prior integration of the research process with the process of policy and decision making.

Box 8.8 The Lothian Five Practice Survey

Objective
Identify need amenable to primary health care intervention.

Process
Survey of patients in five general practices to allow interpractice comparisons to be made. Comparative profiles highlighting significant differences in data from one practice compared with the other four were sent to each of the practices for discussion.

Findings
There were significant differences amongst the practices. *Practice 1* was significantly 'better off' on all but two or three of the measures included in the questionnaire, that is, the socioeconomic circumstances of the practice population were better, the reported morbidity and service use lower, perceived health status was higher and demand for services lower.

Practice 2, in an area of social deprivation, was much worse off in the key areas of psychosocial and mental health and respiratory health. The practice had similar morbidity for ongoing conditions as the 'better-off' practice despite having a significantly younger practice population. The survey also showed that the high use of services was not related to a greater propensity to consult.

Impact
Practice 1. One area of relative unmet need in this practice which the survey did identify was for additional district nursing, an issue which was currently being addressed by the locality. Whilst this practice found the results reassuring, the survey had few implications for service development.

Practice 2. Discussions with the primary health care team focused on the need for a local strategy for mental health.

General. The survey findings have been widely disseminated throughout the area, in particular to the local partnership (a multi-agency organization run by local people) who were in the process of developing their own health strategy. Despite this dissemination, the survey findings have not been translated into a strategy.

Whilst recognizing the strengths of the survey method, particularly for collecting information on people's views and perceptions of health and illness, this study also examined the dangers of developing priorities based on people's opinions taken at face value. The results were analysed to distinguish two different, and often implicit, definitions of need. The analysis showed that popularity of services differed between healthy and unhealthy people, and whilst an interpretation of need based upon popularity may have democratic appeal, it is very different from a definition of need based upon extent of distress. Whilst this analysis of survey data made explicit the difference between equality and equity, the importance of the differing interpretations of need is not confined to this method of collecting people's views and perceptions of need. Other methods, including participatory, qualitative or mixed method approaches, frequently fail to address the crucial issue of equity (Hopton & Dlugolecka 1995).

Operational needs assessments

Four examples of operational needs assessments are described below. They were undertaken to address issues or areas which had been identified for development. They cover a range of topics and integrate a range of methods and data into the process.

The siting of a new service – oncology services in the Wirral

Size. Wirral Health Authority area

Objectives. Plan the expansion of oncology services in the north west of England; to understand the relationship between health needs, service provision, demographic data and environmental conditions in the context of substantial social variations in mortality.

Process. Use of Geographical Information Systems (GIS) to integrate a wide range of data sources which are linked by a geographic or spatial reference, usually the postcode. Several data sets, linked by postcode, were used in the analysis including information from the 1991 census, the regional inpatient information database, sites of current oncology service providers and the clinical information system of the current centre for oncology. The Wirral as a whole was divided into small areas based on the Super-Profile classification system. This system of classifying areas is analogous to the better known ACORN system, and was developed from a cluster analysis of 55 indicators from the 1981 Census Small Area Statistics.

Findings. In the region as a whole, mortality rates for lung cancer for affluent and underprivileged areas vary from less than the national average to nearly three times the national average. The GIS analysis showed that there were large negative differences in the access of under-privileged groups to oncology services and treatments and in the ratio of mortality to morbidity for these groups, suggesting that these two findings were related.

Impact. The research produced two options for the siting of the new service, and allowed decision makers to analyse and choose the best of these options. Wirral Health are actively seeking to redistribute resources to underprivileged areas. The classification combines indicators of the socioeconomic structure of the population with broader lifestyle characteristics (see Table 8.2 for examples).

The organization of inter-professional health needs assessment in two London localities – The London Project

As yet there has been little systematic exploration of the implications of interprofessional working for the process of health needs assessment.

One exception is work carried out in two similar-sized wards of London (Box 8.9). A local multidisciplinary workshop identified health needs assessment as an area

for development and considered the contribution that primary health care teams could make. The potential of patch-based versus practice-based approaches were considered, and the problems of coterminosity and comparability of practice-held versus area-based data highlighted.

A project to address the primary health care needs of a disadvantaged population – The West Central Halifax Project

A project in west Halifax drew on the principles of community development as a basis for what the project described as 'solution orientated health needs assessment' (Box 8.10). The project was funded by an Urban Aid Grant and had its own management structure. The project was based in a small geographical locality of between 11 000 and 12 000 people. The area is one of high deprivation and in which approximately 50% of the population are from south Asian countries. The project focused on the development of primary care, and thus takes a narrower approach than is usual for community development (Ong et al 1991) but is more congruent with the remit of NHS commissioning, which characterizes current locality developments.

The project illustrates well a strategic and politically aware approach rather than one which is methodologically driven. At the outset, the importance of a phenomenological approach to understanding need, and the use of

---

Box 8.9 The London Project

Size of localities
Approximately 7300 people and 2700 households.

Objectives
To identify needs in two similar-sized but apparently different electoral wards chosen to study the contribution that patch-based and practice-based primary care team members could make and the organizational issues of the patch-based needs assessment process. To introduce team working to participants.

Process
An overall patch-based approach was adopted. Both primary health care teams agreed on the data to be collected, and included identifying those receiving state benefits, the proportion of people who were chair bound, with 'significant' disability or on 'at risk' registers, and the proportion of people with asthma. Members of the teams also agreed specific definitions of these terms to ensure the reliability of the data. Teams met regularly to discuss health needs and the development of strategy.

Findings
The project highlighted several important organizational issues. First, how to identify who are the relevant health professionals. For example, approximately 56 GPs had patients in one of the wards, although there were only two practices, each with two partners, within the ward boundaries. Second, different health professionals often had very different views on needs and priorities. Third, participation of small practices was low and this highlighted the particular difficulties that small practices face in becoming actively involved in health needs assessment and commissioning. Finally, the work demonstrated that health needs assessment requires an organizational and management framework as well as a methodological one.

Impact
Professionals learnt much about each other's roles and developed widely networked self-supporting teams beyond their practices. Participants reported it had helped them care better.

Box 8.10 The West Central Halifax Project

Size
A small geographical locality of between 11 000 and 12 000 people.

Objective
The main work areas of the project were to develop interpreting and linkworker services, developing public consultation and advocacy, developing a locality awareness programme for staff, needs and services for the under fives, developing health promotion for south Asian populations in respect of diabetes, coronary heart disease and asthma, developing a neighbourhood health centre, and a specific review of health visiting services as well as a review of other health services.

Process
The project used information and data from a range of sources, including semistructured interviews with at least 80% of those working in primary care settings. They made explicit the dominant elements of project management including devising an accountability structure for the project, using specific management techniques such as matrix management, critical pathing, focusing on finding solutions rather than identifying problems and working up agreed 'exit strategies' to ensure sustainability of developments by bringing them into mainstream service provision.

Impact
Despite the considerable thought and effort which went into public consultation and into understanding the experiences of local people, the project identified difficulties that individuals face in envisaging and articulating service developments.

appropriate methods, was acknowledged. The project used cultural marginalization as its theoretical base, that is that the further the individual's culture is from the culture of the service organization the more difficult the service will be to access and the smaller the likelihood that it will be addressing needs. It is important to remember that the theory of cultural marginalization can refer to women, children, adolescents, the unemployed as well as people from different ethnic cultures, and in that sense it is not identical with the concept of culture as it is used in ordinary language. The project took a multiagency approach and aimed to promote joint working and problem solving.

A project to address the health and social needs of older people – The Salford Elders Project

This project (Box 8.11) uses different types of questionnaire instrument, collects qualitative and quantitative

---

Box 8.11   The Salford Elders Project

Objective
To develop a strategy for improving the health of older people in a single locality.

Process
The project used epidemiological data and the views of professionals and older people themselves in order to identify needs. Initial research was carried out using a semistructured questionnaire administered to 188 local people aged over 65 years to highlight the issues influencing health and well-being, to investigate perceived needs and solutions and to begin an assessment of the priorities of this group.

On the basis of the needs identification, outcomes for what the project was trying to achieve were set. These were to enable older people to make informed choices about available services, to have maximum mobility, to reduce the sense of social isolation and to increase their sense of security inside and outside the home. Options or ideas to address the identified needs were generated by the project task group. All ideas were recorded initially. These were then narrowed to a list of 30 options, and a set of criteria devised by which to appraise the options (see Box 8.4).

In the initial screening of options, priority was given to the views of older people and local workers. A further survey of older people was carried out. The survey presented matched pairs of the generated options and the results analysed to produce a prioritized list of options. Local workers ranked each option on a scale of 1–5. The top 16 options were appraised in terms of the other criteria.

Impact
From each of the options a set of recommendations for specific relevant agencies were developed to form the basis of the strategy. For example, with the option to help relieve people from long-term physical pain came recommendations to commission services differently. This included services for the prevention of osteoporosis and falls, promotion of exercise, increased access to hip replacements and coronary artery bypass grafts, appropriate prescribing of pain relief and referral to secondary care pain relief, and improved access to complementary therapy services. To address the option to increase police in areas with high numbers of older people, recommendations were made to the police service to review existing beat patrols, to extend home watch and community watch schemes and to work with residents, associates and community groups to monitor the services.

---

data. Service uses were involved at all stages of option appraisal.

ASSESSING THE NEEDS FOR RESOURCES

This section considers locality needs assessment in the context of localities as areas for resource allocation and management. Although we have chosen to consider this administrative function of localities separately, the framework for health needs assessment outlined above of purpose, principles and process applies here also. Before we consider these, we give an overview of the context.

The context of locality resource allocation and management

Two key factors shape the context of resource allocation. Firstly, it is important to acknowledge that the politics of what is a sufficient amount of cash to run the NHS (a normative question) is separate from the need to distribute the existing pot of money in an equitable fashion. Resource allocation is thus based on comparative needs assessment; whose relative needs are greater than whose. It is a 'zero-sum' game, one locality's gain will be another's loss.

Secondly, it is important to clarify which resources are being considered and the structure of budgets. As Figure 8.1 indicates, the vast majority of NHS resources (69%) are spent under the cash-limited hospital and community health services (HCHS) budget heading and, on the whole, resource allocation issues are inevitably focused on access to acute and community health services. None

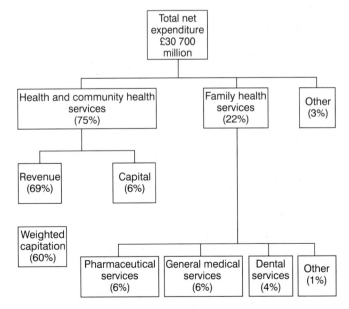

Figure 8.1   Allocation of NHS resources: spending plans for England 1994–95. (From Judge & Mays 1994.)

of the family health services (FHS) budgets is usually taken into account. Despite historically being administratively separate, at the level of service provision they are clearly linked with expenditure from one budget offsetting another and all are subject to 'cost-shifting'.

Acknowledging these links and integrating these budgets remains an important issue for the policy thrust of the market and the moves towards a primary care-led NHS.

The purpose and principles of resource allocation

As with other forms of needs assessment, assessment of need for resource allocation must consider the purpose and principles. In particular, is equity the core principle or are there other policy issues to consider? If equity is an important aim, how are we to achieve it. For instance, is it:

- Equalizing cash per head for health care delivery (based on expected need and capacity to benefit)?
- Equality in the use of/access to health services?
- Equalizing health status?

Some are more related to 'needs' than others. All will produce different processes and results.

For most administrative purposes, equity of resource inputs, or equalizing cash per head, is the most practical objective to pursue. In this context, there are three issues at the core of resource allocation:

- What are the current budgets?
- What should the budgets be?
- How do we reduce inequities (how do we get budgets to their 'correct' level)?

Ultimately all budgets are developed from an historical base. The extent to which historical budgets are equitable or related to need is questionable. For example, historical budgets are based on level of service provision, which in turn has implications for demand, though service provision and demand are not necessarily related to need.

There has been much policy debate on how to adjust budgets to take account of unmet need or unexpressed demand. If the current distribution of resources is not equitable how do we define what is fair and how, in practical terms, can resources be shifted to their most equitable distribution and how can localities, sublocality areas or practices adjust the level of service demand accordingly (Sheldon et al 1991)?

Methods and process of resource allocation

In this section we review methods and processes of resource allocation and their relationship to the principles outlined above. Four methods are described:

- Historically based budgets
- Benchmarking
- The use of ad hoc resources
- The development and use of formulas.

Historically based budgets

In principle, setting historically based budgets is straightforward. The basic steps are:

- Identify NHS activity by locality (episodes in hospitals/contacts in the community)
- Identify an appropriate cost base (GPFH procedure prices from local providers, for instance)
- Multiply the two to get a budget figure.

In practice, however, there are major problems with data. The shortcomings of NHS episode data have been discussed elsewhere. A further complicating factor is the inaccuracy of the hospital cost base. Most hospitals do not know what it costs to provide their services. Budgets based on local prices could mean major adjustments to budgets that have been set in previous years. Further still, collecting baseline data is problematic for two reasons. First, use of historical data serves to perpetuate inefficient practice. For example, GPs that currently 'buy' inpatient care when a day case procedure is available will have no incentive to change their practice as they receive more funds for the inpatient work. Second, during the initial period of data collection it is possible for referrals to hospitals to be 'inflated' in order to affect the budget level to be set.

Benchmarking

Benchmarking is being promoted by the Department of Health partially as a way of getting around the problems of historical budget setting. Benchmarking is a comparative process which assesses service level activity adjusted for several factors including the age and sex distribution of the population concerned. They are derived by multiplying average activity rates (norms) by the practice population. Activity 'norms' are produced at regional level for application to local populations (DOH 1994). Ultimately, though, benchmarking is no more than a sophisticated adjunct to historically based budget setting.

Ad hoc monies and bidding

A bidding system for resource allocation would have some advantages, though possibly even greater disadvantages. On the plus side, it is relatively simple, and money can be targeted to priorities. The disadvantages are that bidding is time-consuming, frustrating, and potentially inequitable (localities with good bid writers are likely to attract the most resources). Whilst bidding processes would not be appropriate for the allocation of all resources to localities, it would allow for a degree of central strategic direction on the part of the district health authorities. Marginal (top-sliced) resources can be used to target specific areas of need to achieve specific outcomes. How far this would be politically acceptable to the new generation of GP commissioners has not been tested.

The use of formulas

The use of formulas offers the opportunity to promote equity by including weighting factors. Two approaches can be taken:

1. Using 'off-the-shelf' weighting factors
2. Developing your own method/weightings.

Each has advantages and disadvantages. Regardless of the option taken, there are three basic steps to any formula for resource allocation:

Step 1: weight for age, younger and older age groups use health services to a greater extent than other age groups and therefore 'cost' more on the average.
Step 2: weight for need (discussed below).
Step 3: weight for market forces, or the legitimate differentials in the cost of resource inputs.

Age weightings, representing the average spend per head of population in each age group, are readily available for use (NHS Executive 1994). Localities could develop their own age weightings if local prices were felt to be more relevant than national figures. Market forces are used to correct for the differential cost of inputs (land, capital and labour) across the country, but this is less likely to be a significant factor at the locality level (even in London).

Most of the debate about weighting centres on the weighting for need, in particular how to operationalize the concept of need in terms of routinely available data given that there are few data on morbidity which are independent of service use. The link between socioeconomic status and morbidity and ill-health suggests that data on socioeconomic status or deprivation which are routinely available could be used as a proxy indicator of need.

Even within this approach there is no agreement on which factors in the available data truly reflect need in communities. For example, there are three well-known indices for deprivation – Carstairs and Morris (1989), Townsend et al (1988) and Jarman (1983). There are also the recently developed needs weighting factors from York University (Carr-Hill et al 1994) that are in the new Department of Health formula. The latter is based on a model that takes into account the previous use of health services and their costs. (See Table 8.4 for comparison of the elements included.)

The sources of information on needs used in formulas are routine datasets such as the Public Health Common Dataset (for mortality), the census and health service activity. The weighting factors in the York model were derived by combining all three. It is possible to apply these weightings to locality populations because the base data are routinely available. The drawback of this approach is that not all need may be reflected in usage. Indeed, Sheldon's work on a formula for GPFH procedures indicated that higher socioeconomic status groups appear to have greater access to services.

Alternative weightings to the York formula could be

Table 8.4 Variables included in deprivation indices

Variable	Carstairs	Jarman	Townsend	York (Acute)	York (Psychiatric)
Unemployment	✓	✓	✓	✓	
No car	✓		✓		
Low social class	✓				
Unskilled		✓			
Overcrowding	✓	✓	✓		
Not owner occupied			✓		
Single parent		✓	✓		✓
Under age 5 years		✓			
Lone pensioners		✓		✓	✓
1 year immigrants		✓			
Ethnic minorities		✓			
SMR>75				✓	✓
SIR				✓	
Single carer households				✓	
People born in New Commonwealth					✓
Permanent sick rates					✓
Dependants in no carer households					✓

Adapted from Morris & Carstairs (1991).
SMR, standardized mortality rate for the under 75 year olds; SIR, standardized illness ratio for the 0–74 year age range.

any of the other deprivation indices already mentioned, or just using mortality as a proxy for ill-health (e.g. SMR>75).

Understandably, local areas feel their circumstances require a different process of weighting to reflect local factors. Before embarking on developing local weightings for need there are three crucial considerations:

1. Derivation from a consensus of those who will be affected by the policy is needed. Local agreement on the important factors to use as weightings should be obtained.
2. Simplicity is essential for practical application, and that will inevitably require compromises.
3. Some 'face' validity is essential. The areas with 'acknowledged' deprivation should have this reflected in the weightings.

It is important to bear in mind that formulas only describe an optimal position if resources were distributed equitably. The problem of how to reach this position remains. The process of formula development outlined above should help to defuse arguments with those that will inevitably be losers. Districts with substantial growth monies may find this relatively easier than those who have limited or no growth in finances. Growth monies allow a levelling-up process to be undertaken, i.e. holding the funds of 'over-target' practices at the same level in real terms. Levelling down – actually taking resources away – will be politically very difficult, but its impact will have to be carefully considered.

The approach taken by North Derbyshire (North Derbyshire Health 1995) considers these issues, and explicitly addresses the question of 'what is equitable?' and how to achieve equity.

North Derbyshire have initiated a 2% policy whereby over/under-target practices are moved towards their target at a rate of 2% per year (so a practice at 110% of target would take 5 years to reach equity). Importantly, they have developed a set of principles upon which this policy stands. These are as follows:

● A levelling-up approach would not be sufficient (over-target practices must release resources)
● GPs must perceive the benefits of redistribution
● The health authority must be able to present proper stewardship of resources (accountability and responsibility)
● Long-term spending patterns should not be changed too quickly
● Spending targets must be indicative only
● Over-target practices will need active support in achieving change
● Under-target practices also need support to move towards their target
● The formula should be reviewed at regular intervals.

This begs the question of how resources are managed at the locality level in relation to need. Localities and practices will face two pressures:

1. A fixed limit on the resources they are able to use (defined by broad concepts of need, i.e. deprivation and death)
2. A welter of information on the 'actual' needs of the locality/community (based on normative needs assessment).

Techniques will need to be used/developed to manage the potential dissonance between the two. These will apply to those gaining resources as well as those losing them (two of North Derbyshire's principles).

One possible technique is 'marginal analysis', mentioned above in the context of option appraisal. This economic technique starts from the position that service changes are made on the 'margin' or incrementally. The principle is *nothing much will change but what does change is important*. From this perspective, marginal analysis can be seen as putting Charles Lindblom's 'science of muddling through' (Lindblom 1959) onto a rational and explicit basis. This will clearly reflect the position of localities who, as in the case of North Derbyshire, may face changes in their budgets of around 2% per year.

CONCLUSION AND DISCUSSION

Different localities have developed different corporate structures, functions, interests, resources and ideologies, and this diversity makes a 'how to do it' approach to locality health needs assessment inappropriate. This chapter has therefore taken an analytical approach which has considered the purpose, principles and process of health needs assessments in order to guide decisions about health needs assessments in specific locality settings or across localities in a district.

The chapter has argued that thinking about the purpose, principles and process of health needs assessment is essential to identify appropriate research, development or managerial methods and to link health needs assessments with locality functions and the commissioning process. Where an assessment is planned at a locality level, considerable care should be taken to design an appropriate process and use methods which are valid, reliable and appropriate to the stage of the health needs assessment process. An important and frequently neglected issue is acknowledging that 'methods' of health needs assessments are not value-free. Only by making the principles and values explicit can they be recognized and negotiated.

The new impetus for locality planning within the NHS has arisen in response to the problems of fragmentation and inequity inherent in GPFH. However, the tension between fragmentation of district strategy and local sensitivity remains, and part of negotiating this tension is the consideration of the appropriate functions of localities and the wider debate about the limits and potential of a locality approach to health care planning. Developing an effective combination of confederation and subsidiarity may be required. For health needs assessment this means considering which needs are best assessed at the individual general practice level, which at the locality level, and which require district wide assessment. Some localities may be too small or too large to support some methods, and broad-based needs assessments focusing on small geographic areas may inevitably tend to neglect important minority groups and health problems for which a district wide strategy may be required. Equally it may be inefficient to replicate similar needs assessments in localities across a district. From the case studies reviewed here, operational needs assessments to develop service delivery or initiatives in an identified priority area for which resources have been allocated appear to be most congruent with a locality approach.

The chapter has side-stepped two further important and interrelated issues: the relationship between health services, personal and social services and wider socio-political change and the enduring problem of linking health needs assessments to resource allocation and resource management. Whilst localities have long been seen as a focus for interagency and intersectoral cooperation, it is unclear whether and how the current NHS localities based on general practices will coordinate resource management and service development with local authority personal and social services to seek solutions outside the health sector.

Given the dilemmas and ambiguities of locality health needs assessment, and health needs assessment generally (Salter 1993), it is important to ask whether it is a worthwhile endeavour that leads to change other than a means of giving legitimacy to prior decisions and the credibility of commissioners. There are important arguments that the process of health needs assessment can be of value in developing teamwork, introducing individuals involved to each other and to ideas or issues that may eventually lead to change within or outwith the commissioning process. The approach taken in this chapter is open to the criticism that it is naive to imply that the commissioning process or locality functions 'exist' or can be defined with any clarity. In this context, health needs assessment may be of heuristic value in critically reflecting on the commissioning process and locality functions. The question remains as to whether health needs assessment is the most appropriate means of tackling these issues.

BIBLIOGRAPHY

Bradshaw J 1972 A taxonomy of social need. In: McLachlan G (ed) Problems and progress in medical care. Oxford University Press, London

Bullen N, Moon G, Jones K 1996 Defining localities for health planning: a GIS approach. Social Science and Medicine 309: 781–784

Burrage H 1994 Epidemiology and community health: a strained connection. Social Science and Medicine 25: 895–903

Canning S 1994 Report pulls its punches on nursing's role in purchasing. Nursing Standard 8: 5

Cohen D 1994 Marginal analysis in practice: an alternative to needs assessment for contracting healthcare. British Medical Journal 309: 781–784

Cohen G, Forbes J, Garraway M 1995 Interpreting self reported limiting long term illness. British Medical Journal 311: 722–724

Department of Health 1989 Working for patients. HMSO, London

Donabedian A 1993 Aspects of medical care administration. Harvard University Press, Cambridge, MA

Fettes J 1994 Joint contracting and development project. Report for the Scottish Office Management Executive

Gaffy J P, Williams J 1994 Purchasing for all: an alternative to fundholding. British Medical Journal 308: 391–394

Ham C 1992 Locality purchasing, discussion paper 30. Health Services Management Centre, University of Birmingham

Hopton J L, Dlugolecka M 1995a Patient's perceptions of need for primary health care services: useful for priority setting? British Medical Journal 310: 1237–1240

Hopton J L, Dlugolecka M 1995b Need and demand for primary health care: a comparative survey approach. British Medical Journal 310: 1369–1373

Judge K, Mays N 1994 British Medical Journal 308: 1363–1366

Kitsuse J I, Spector M 1973 Toward a sociology of social problems: social conditions, value-judgements and social problems. Social Problems 20: 407–419

MacIntyre S, MacIver S, Sooman A 1993 Area, class and health: should we be focusing on places or people? Journal of Social Policy 22: 213–234

Meethan K, Thompson C 1993 Politics, locality and resources: negotiating a community care scheme. Policy and Politics 21: 195–205

Milburn K, Fraser E, Secker J, Pavis S 1995 Combining methods in health promotion research: some considerations about appropriate use. Health Education Journal 54: 347–356

Moon G 1990 Conceptions of space and community in British health policy. Social Science and Medicine 30: 165–171

Morley V 1993 Empowering GPs as purchasers. British Medical Journal 306: 112–114

National Association of Commissioning Groups 1995 Cohesion: the contribution of GP commissioning groups to the development of a primary care led NHS. National Association of Commissioning Groups

Ong B N, Humphris G, Annett H, Rifkin S 1991 Rapid appraisal in an urban setting, an example from the developed world. Social Science and Medicine 32: 909–915

Plampling D, Delamothe T 1991 The citizen's charter and the NHS. British Medical Journal 303: 203–204

Popay J, Williams G (eds) 1994 Researching the people's health. Routledge, London

Porter M, MacIntyre S 1994 What is must be best: a research note on conservative or deferential responses to antenatal care provision. Social Science and Medicine 19: 1197–1200

Salter B 1993 The politics of purchasing in the NHS. Policy and Politics 21: 171–184

Sheldon T A, Davey Smith G, Bevan G 1991 Weighting in the dark: resource allocation in the new NHS. British Medical Journal 306: 835–839

Todd P B J, Brown P 1994 The demography of demand for oncology services: a healthcare planning GIS application. Health and Emergency Services

Twigg, L 1990 Health based geographical information systems: their potential examined in the light of existing data sources. Social Science and Medicine 30: 143–155

Wainwright D 1996 The best of both worlds. Health Service Journal, 25 Jan

Winkler F 1987 Consumerism in healthcare; beyond a supermarket model. Policy and Politics 15: 1–8

Young K, Haynes R 1993 Assessing population needs in primary health care: the problem of GP attachment. Journal of Interprofessional Care 7: 15–27

APPENDIX

Reviewed needs assessments and case studies*

Barking and Havering Health Authority. Keynes H February 1995. Health and social profiles of localities: locality 4 DPH research report No 40–4 of locality reports for primary care. Directorate of Public Health, Romford

* Bexley and Greenwich Health 1995 Locality development plans 1995/96: Eltham locality. Bexley and Greenwich Health, London

Bradford Health Reports 1 and 2. , Boswell C 1995 GP's role in commissioning health

East Kent Project. Burnett A C 1995 Locality commissioning in East Kent – a project contributing to the development of primary care-led purchasing. Unpublished

Healthy Eastender's Project 1994. Fair Shares in health care. Preliminary Report, Queen Mary and Westfield College, London

Leicestershire Health. *Jennings S 1995 West central Halifax primary health care project. Leicester

London project. *Singer R G 1992 Primary care teams and the needs assessment process: a report on sabbatical leave and its associated project. London

Lothian Health Survey. Cohen G, Forbes J, Garraway M 1995 Final report. Department of Public Health Sciences, University of Edinburgh, Edinburgh; *Hopton J, Dlugolecka M 1996 Assessment of health needs applicable to primary care: the development of a general practice based model. Final report to the Scottish Office CSO

Salford Elders Project. *Williamson I, Popay J, Cohen Z 1994 Salford locality health needs assessment project: the needs of older people. Report. Salford & Trafford Health Authorities

West Central Halifax Primary Health Care Project. *Kelly T 1995. West Yorkshire Health Authority

Wirral. *Todd P B J, Brown P 1994 The demography of demand for oncology services: a healthcare planning GIS application. Health and Emergency Services

* Denotes case study

REFERENCES & COMMENTS

British Cardiac Society 1994 Council statement on the demand and need for cardiac services and the development of a waiting list strategy for cardiac disease

Carr-Hill R A, Hardman G, Martin S, Peacock S, Sheldon T, Smith P 1994 A formula for distributing NHS revenues based on small area use of hospital beds. Centre for Health Economics University of York

Carstairs V, Morris R 1989 Deprivation and mortality: an alternative to social class? Community Medicine 11: 210–219

Clarke A, McKee M 1995 Guidelines, enthusiasms, uncertainty and the limits to purchasing. British Medical Journal 310: 101–104,

Department of Health 1984 EL(94)84 General Practice Fundholding: Guidance on setting budgets for 1995/96

Healthy Eastenders Project 1994 Fair shares in health care preliminary report. Queen Mary and Westfield College, London

Jarman B 1983 Identification of underprivileged areas. British Medical Journal 286: 1705–1708

Judge K, Mays N 1994 British Medical Journal 308: 1363–1366

Lindblom C E 1959 The 'Science of Muddling Through' Public Administration Review (Spring)

NHS Executive 1994 HCHS revenue capitation allocation: weighted capitation formula, Leeds

North Derbyshire Health 1995 Final Report of the North Derbyshire Equity Group

Morris R, Carstairs V 1991 Deprivation and Health in Scotland, Aberdeen University Press

Townsend P, Phillimore P, Beattie A 1988 Health and Deprivation: inequality and the North London: Croom Helm

9

The role of community trusts

Laurann Yen   Liz Haggard

Why would community health trusts, or trusts of any kind, want to invest time and money in needs assessment when one of the key planks of the National Health Service (NHS) reforms has been the cementing of the commissioner's, and in particular the public health department's, role in identifying needs and making commissioning and purchasing decisions on behalf of their local residents? Does a community health trust have a role in needs assessment within a primary care-led NHS where much of the decision making will occur within primary health care teams? Does needs assessment take valuable time and energy away from the development of the provider role, or is it fundamental to the 'good health' of a provider organization?

This chapter proposes that community health trusts are, and should be, involved in needs assessment at a number of levels, contributing both to good purchasing decisions, and good providing decisions influencing the end outcome for the user. It also provides examples of ways in which community health trusts are involved in needs assessment, and the changes this can bring about in health care. In an NHS without a formal contracting system, the potential community trust role is even greater.

The rationale for community trusts undertaking needs assessments includes:

- *Good practice.* Professionals working in health services believe that they have a responsibility to identify patient need in order to ensure that the most appropriate service is sought to enable those needs to be met.
- *Corporate effectiveness.* Contracting systems are often 'blunt' and differentially developed, offering, certainly in primary and community health care services, a relatively non-specific outline of expected services. The provider trust must make many of the decisions about 'how' a contract will be met, refining the contracting specification to a delivery of service

within the parameters of its financial and skills portfolio. An involvement in needs assessment is required to develop a successful reconciliation between the strategic and operational demands in the trust.

- *Changing practice.* The contracting process may initiate change in services, but the capacity to make change at the rate and level which would match the potential will be limited by the resources available to enter the debate, and by the priority placed on their importance – changes to service are likely to occur at the margins, and need to be informed through clinical practice intelligence which is held within provider services. In reality, the effectiveness of contract changes depends on the prior commitment and practice changes of clinical staff.
- *Influencing commissioning decisions.* Trusts have an interest in developing services for both organizational and consumer benefit, and must ensure that they are able to influence the contracting process through offering alternatives and potential developments to the commissioner. Reconfiguring a portfolio of existing services within current budgets is often the only available means of service development. It critically depends on providers identifying feasible opportunities. In a primary care-led NHS, commissioning general practices will need to be offered such options.

Table 9.1 offers a view which takes us from the assessment of need to the delivery of service, identifying roles within each component of the health structure.

The assessment of need at the population level which forms the basis for commissioning, and purchasing decisions will be translated into direct care by the provider organization, the hands on care-giver and by the interaction between the care-giver and the client. This translation will be shaped by:

- The *evidence* available to support the usefulness/efficacy of the care thought to be needed – one of the tensions within health/social care is around the various options which might be available to meet the same need, and the shift to evidence-based purchasing reflects the need to create an open debate.

- The *public acceptance* of the proposed care – will the community accept the purchasing decision, even if the basis for the decision appears sound in health terms?
- The *professional view* of the care professional will have a very strong influence in defining health and health issues, with the capacity to define needs and the potential responses the service could make. Examples might include roles and jobs which used to be associated only with doctors, which are now increasingly in the domain of nursing and other professional staff, shifting the definitions of health and social care, changing policies on good practice. An analysis of the different care provided by entering the 'care' system at different points offers good illustrations of this, with 'need' often determined by a professionally centred, rather than by a client centred, approach.
- *Political support* for the care – not just for the political 'noise' which the choice might create, but for the philosophy of the decision and who pays.
- *Cost and predicted duration* of care, which is crucial for primary care and community health services where their involvement in the care of individual clients and in communities tends to be ongoing, and at times relatively diffuse.

Information passes to the commissioning organization through the same provider channels, and will be similarly influenced, so that it will be an amalgam of client expressed need and professional and organizational provider views.

When commissioners want to make changes in the pattern of services they commission, there needs to be a reconciliation between developing access to new services and honouring existing commitments (accrual). These commitments may, for example in the case of care of chronic illness, be long term. Then the portfolio of services which end up being delivered may not appear to be cohesive and planned. Additionally, the need to precommit resources over a long period will limit opportunities for 'new' services, will create tension between the proponents of each decision, and may well be the cause

Commissioning	Provider – organization	Provider – care-giver
assess need – health and social	market services – current and new	work to contract – on quality and cost
review effectiveness evidence	accept contract	– on quality and cost
direct puchasing intentions in light of resources	train staff to work to contract	predict pattern and length of care
select providers	monitor individual care, contract compliance and unmet need	identify unmet/overmet need for both individuals and community
monitor individual and population need		

Table 9.1

of much of the frustration felt by care providers (and purchasers). Continuous assessment of need is fundamental to the capacity to direct resources into the appropriate areas, even where resources are to a large extent pre-committed to ongoing care requirements.

If community health trusts take needs assessment seriously, in looking at:

- Good practice
- Corporate need
- Changing clinical practice
- Influencing purchasing decisions,

they will achieve:

- More effective services
- Better targeting of resources
- Better fit between the expressed intentions of the commissioning organization and the service portfolio of the provider organization
- Better market understanding and a stronger market position.

GOOD PRACTICE

Working out how best to be involved in the assessment of need has been a particular issue for community health services, where the commitment to identifying and responding to the needs of populations, both small and large, has been so much part of the culture of their professions and organizations.

The fundamental contribution community health trusts make to needs assessment is the knowledge and professional assessment of staff providing direct care. Many purchasers acknowledge the value of incorporating the 'grass roots' knowledge of the community health and primary care professionals. In seeking access to general practitioner (GP) held practice information, purchasers have tried to use a body of information to formulate their purchasing intentions. There has always been an issue over access to, and use of, community health services information because of the diffuse and non-comparable way in which it is collected and interpreted. Proper involvement of these services in contributing the practitioner perspective to population or group needs assessment has been weaker than it ought to be.

The model used in Chiswick, outlined in detail later in this chapter, offers the use of the Community Minimum Data Set as a way of creating a confidential, multisite, multipractitioner information set which describes current activity and enables decisions to come from a clear knowledge of both morbidity and service activity.

Within primary health care teams, many community health staff are involved in developing their individual practice profiles, or in contributing to the profile of the general practice or locality in which they work. This is particularly the case in health visiting, where the development of a profile of practice is integral to good practice, but is becoming increasingly the case in other branches of community nursing. The profile typically sets out practice population characteristics, some information about the locality and some figures indicating the number of patients with particular conditions in the practice population, which creates a basic indication of likely need. The recent requirement for general practices to produce an annual report has increased practices' interest in practice profiles. The contributions of health visitors have, on the whole, been welcome. In Shipley, for example, there is a contract between a practice and the local trust for the collection of practice profiling data. In the Castlefields practice in Runcorn, the needs assessment work done initially through a project was intended to transfer to the responsibility of health visitors, but it was thought that the work was properly the remit of the whole primary health care team (Colin-Thomé, 1996 Castlefields Fundholding Model).

The danger of this kind of profile is that it tends to stand alone and will reflect the quality of the data available. Without comparative data to show if 10 patients with breast cancer in the practice are more or less than expected, or statistical information to help assess whether this is a random fluctuation, the profile information is too uncertain for any action to be taken. However, if comparative information is available, perhaps from public health specialists, the fact that the practice as a whole shares the profile information may make it more likely that a balanced judgement can be made of the figures, and changes and interventions will be agreed. For example, a practice which finds that it has higher than expected levels of asthma might set up an asthma clinic at the treatment end of the practice response, or at the prevention end might search for possible aspects of life in the community linked to increased asthma and try to secure changes.

This approach has been put into place in the Limehouse practice in Tower Hamlets, where concerns over the level of respiratory illness in the practice and local population have led to a broad-based assessment of need involving community health staff, GPs, the local authority and local community organizations. It was clear from this assessment that much of the burden of illness resulted from poor environmental conditions and poverty, which has contributed to the development of housing clinics and a multi-agency energy efficiency project.

The health visitor, working as part of the Stepney Nursing Development Unit, has been a driving force within the project and demonstrates the powerful public health role which can be fulfilled by these professionals. This represents 'good practice' in the wide sense, and will enable a more effective and powerful intervention, at both individual and community levels than one which addresses only the 'disease' and not the cause.

The 'micro-purchasing' project in Yorkshire (West & Poulton 1995) used needs assessment to develop profiles to determine the allocation of clinical resources within the broad primary health care team. Community Trust staff across 10 sites worked with their general practitioners to:

- Jointly identify need within their practice populations
- Work through a planning process to identify the most appropriate use of resources
- Make the changes required to match more effectively the needs of the client groups with the skills and resources available to the team
- Make decisions about changing the structure of the team
- Develop different skills portfolios
- Change the balance of service provided.

The assessment of individual need remains the fundamental approach used with Community Health Trusts. This assessment will determine the care plan for each client, and the continuing assessment of each client's need will ensure that, as needs change, service input changes to meet them.

In many cases, the professional assessment of need complements the expressed needs of the service user. Part of the skill in assessment consists of looking beyond the subjective view of the service user, often coloured by fear and anxiety, to identify the real changing need. For example, where someone is terminally ill, they or their carers and family may feel that they need the support of a high-technology environment – community health trusts can often provide an opportunity to assess and meet a wider and more holistic need for the client and family. Community trusts can ensure that the crucial information about existing and potential need is heard within the commissioning structure. They need to develop better ways of creating the link between individual assessment and contracts, particularly over time. There is little evidence that current contracts are able to give adequate recognition to changing need profiles, and so they are unable to make meaningful resource shifts to match them. This becomes particularly an issue in the emphasis on 'shifting care from secondary to primary care' where the rhetoric is not backed by research to identify the shifts or implications made, for example, in identifying the additional demands placed on both primary care and community health service (Thomasson 1995).

CORPORATE ISSUES

Community health trusts will use needs assessment to address market analysis, efficiency and cost effective-

ness, monitoring preventative care programmes, investment in skills development and to see opportunities for development.

Marketing

Community health trusts, like other NHS organizations, generally want to develop their services in ways which reconcile the 'social' with the 'business' issues. While they will wish to consolidate and expand their organizational position, developments are also based on the perceived social benefit of the resulting services. Their work promotes the development of services to people at home, identifying potential services or new ways of providing services. Community health trusts use needs assessment, both in attempting to translate the needs of individual clients into contract specifications, and in bidding for resources to support an increasing demand from primary care and community health services. This will be directed to commissioners and GPs, and the need to develop collaborative assessment models which bridge the professional approaches would be well placed within community trusts and primary care.

Efficiency and cost-effectiveness

Community trusts are subject to the same requirements to deliver cost efficiencies as other NHS organizations, and often to create developmental funding from existing contract resources (Thomasson 1995). This will mean that new services, development and the ability to maintain existing services are funded from recycling resources within primary and community health care.

Efficiency and cost effectiveness are both addressed through a continuous assessment of the level of need and the level of required skill and ensuring that the individual user has access to the service required at the level required as needs change.

The work on pressure sore management from York (Effective Health Care, 1995) shows that there is still little consensus on the best way forward for both assessment methodology and management, and a need for more rigorous research to provide 'reliable evidence on the relative cost effectiveness of different strategies'. However, there is a growing body of nurse generated information which is beginning to identify both clinical and cost effectiveness measures and approaches (Rashid, 1995).

The changing provision of family planning services, once very much the domain of community health trusts but increasingly provided within general practice, also reflects these shifts. No real assessment of need has taken place to determine whether or not this represents the best service, but with the targets for cervical smears in place for General Practice, it is almost inevitable that other elements of contraceptive care and advice will be provided within this setting. Community trusts have responded to this by reducing the number of general family planning clinics they offer, and targeting services more towards groups whose needs do not appear to be being met through GP services. This shift may reduce the breadth of needs assessment and, therefore, the potential to provide an appropriate set of services because of an assumption that registration with a GP practice will automatically enable clients to get the service they need. This may discriminate against groups least likely to be able to negotiate the system and obtain good GP services.

The same process is occurring within community children's services, and services reshaped to reflect the changing balance of services. The flexibility that community health trusts show in responding appropriately to these shifts will determine to a large extent their success as provider organizations.

Monitoring preventative care programmes

Applying cost-effectiveness measures to preventative care programmes is fraught with difficulties, but the shift of activity to general practice creates an opportunity for collaborative work. Designing and implementing processes of monitoring screening and surveillance, which consider their impact on population need, would not only be of public health importance, but create new opportunities for community trust staff. These are in training, quality assurance, audit and niche provision. Many trusts are involved in monitoring child health surveillance, and some immunization or cervical screening, often in conjunction with former Family Health Services Authority (FHSA) departments. New health authorities are likely to want to contract out such work.

At a simple, operational level, monitoring the denominator of a screened population is crucial to interpret correctly the coverage figure. This is easier now computerized records are in more common usage, but incorrect data entry and high patient mobility create problems. Table 9.2 illustrates an audit of community trust health visitor caseload against the FHSA record for a non-computerized small general practice. Although the total list size of both health visitors and practice were identical, variations from the corrected denominator population were huge – health visitor caseload by 22%, FHSA list by 15% and practice manual age sex register by 2.5%. Thus, monitoring the population for which the general practice and community trust staff have responsibility is a basic need, which should be built into the working practices of professionals and their activity reports.

Community trust child health departments are well aware of the variation in performance of child health surveillance and immunization against general practices.

	HV caseload	FHSA list	
Children on HV list not on FHSA list	398	448	Children on FHSA list not on HV list
		25	Children inside HV catchment area
		18	Children outside HV catchment area
		−18	Children known to HV as having left register
	−1	−35	Erroneous DOB
Chidren living in B & B	−30		
Children thought registered but left	−12		
With other GP	−1		
Registered according to age/sex register		2	
	397	397	

Variation from corrected denominator population 22% vs 15%

Table 9.2 Audit of under 5 population in small non-computerized general practice (Andrew Harris) with high patient mobility

A study in Glasgow (Lynch 1995) showed that practices with past low uptake rates have a low probability of reaching high targets, and tend to have low child health surveillance and be in maximally deprived areas. There may be scope for community trusts to offer professional and managerial support to these practices, or even bid for a primary care training contract. To make the case, assessing the need of these populations may be an important initial exercise, which should be welcomed by practices whose improved performance would attract the financial benefits of reaching a higher target.

It has been known for a long while that difficulties with appointment times and access to a choice of sites are barriers to uptake of cervical screening. Monitoring of the acceptability of choice and uptake are important, and the findings may generate a case to support a community clinic.

Usually the measure of performance used is coverage (percentage immunized and screened), but that in itself may not be adequate as a measure of need, nor will it indicate how to improve performance.

There is a fear in some districts that non-attenders have a disproportionally high disease risk, and a tool for risk targeting in cervical cancer has been developed (Wilkinson et al 1992). It used educational level, current smoking habit, years of oral contraceptive use and number of sexual partners. This could form the basis of a screening monitoring process, if data were opportunistically recorded on all eligible attendees.

The Cancer Research Campaign Study (Orbell et al 1995) population did not have an epidemiologically higher risk in non-attenders, but did have a higher non-attendance in lower social classes who reported disproportionally higher anxiety and embarrassment at attendance. Risk assessment by women took insufficient consideration of smoking habit; suggesting the value of invitations guiding personal risk assessment. Incorporating strategies into service design which reduce user uncertainty and address the reluctance of women used to dependency may be appropriate. Sophisticated qualitative monitoring of users, non-attenders and providers of local well-women services, based on such findings, is a legitimate needs assessment, which is within the domain of community trusts. It may require public health specialist advice at the design and analysis stages.

Investment in skills development

Alongside the efficiency and effectiveness imperatives lies the need to ensure that the skills which are being developed within community health trusts are appropriate to enable contracts and future plans to be realized. Having established an understanding of the nature of the need within the community, the trusts must look at whether or not this is an area in which they will provide a service, and how they will do so in the most effective and efficient way. The development of nursing skills to cover a wider range of traditionally doctor-provided services, the development of health care assistants, and the capacity to provide more intensive and complex care to people at home are all areas in which investment in new skills is central to successful change.

Community health trusts need to be able to identify where changes in clinical practice will enable more effective services to be provided, and use needs assessment to point to a range of service options which might be provided to meet the needs of individual clients. This fresh look at needs assessment becomes more important as conventional ways of addressing need come under increasing pressure through issues such as shortages in certain professional groups, changing beliefs about effective approaches and the acknowledgement of overlaps in professional boundaries and knowledge bases. This approach challenges the dominance of service, based on 'what is available', and offers one which is more directed to assessing and meeting the needs of the client from a pool of skills and resources. One example of this is the changing approach to meeting acute mental health needs, where a client who would traditionally be assessed in an accident and emergency department by an SHO, may be seen now by an experienced psychiatric nurse or a clinical psychologist, who can provide a much more effective and confident first intervention.

Similarly, the change in the provision of school health services has identified the potential for a range of new services to be offered by nurses, including health assessments and immunizations, which has the potential to alter the balance between the work of community medical officers and school nurses, as well as between general practitioners and community health services.

These shifts are often generated through a need to reassess current practice because of the difficulty in providing services through traditional routes – without knowledge and reassessment of need at both individual and population levels, changes and development of good practice will happen in an ad hoc and inconsistent way, and may never develop the capacity to inform and promote better decision making at either individual or community levels.

A familiar area in primary health care is the changing work of district and practice nurses, and, in the near future, the reshaping of community nursing knowledge and skills through the Post-Registration Education Project. As the Yorkshire work, mentioned earlier, shows, once needs have been established, and primary health care teams are identifying and allocating resources on the basis of need and effectiveness, there can be a shift in the way services are set up and provided. An opportunity is created for direct providers to explore and use both specific profession-based skills, and areas of overlap. The Tower Hamlets review of young disabled services led by an attached public health physician is pointing to the need for a flexible mixed inpatient/day care disabled unit and customized intensive rehabilitation packages of care to promote independent living. Here is an opportunity for leading service development and bidding for new business. (See case study Tower Hamlets Young Rehabilitation Review.)

Community health services are beginning to create 'tailor-made' training to match 'tailor-made' care, developing skills as they are required, or 'just in time' for the care of individual clients. For example, the needs of individual clients are assessed in the 'hospital aftercare' service within the Tower Hamlets health care trust, with a care plan to be followed by the health care assistants providing service, but, where necessary, being given the training they will need to fulfil the plan for each individual client.

However, there is a point at which a 'critical mass' of need is reached, and it becomes clear that training in a particular knowledge or skill is required throughout a clinical area. Community trusts cannot make an appropriate and effective set of training investments without understanding well the needs, both current and potential, of their user population.

INFLUENCING PURCHASING AND PRACTICE – CASE STUDIES

The Chiswick study – Julie Dent

Objective. Ealing Hammersmith and Hounslow Health Agency, setting out to study ways to commission services for care groups within the community, piloted a model in Chiswick using the Community Contracts Minimum Data Set (CCMDS) as the basis for assessing needs and determining service provision and resource allocation across care group needs within a defined population.

Process. The use of CCMDS both enables and requires the provider to be integrally involved in the determination of the data collected, its analysis and in the subsequent discussion with both health commissioning and GP purchasers on future contracting requirements, developing a model of collaborative commissioning firmly based in current activity.

The model used the capacity of the CCMDS to provide information on service referrals within and across service groups and providers. It has particular relevance in establishing the basis for continuous assessment of need through the capacity which emerges to create an interactive data base of client need, service response and the effectiveness of that response, since the system contains all elements on a client-based file which can be built up to give a profile of the client's interaction with the system. At the same time, the potential to cross over needs groups or resource groups allows a more comprehensive picture to be made of the aggregated needs of the broader population served by the community trust.

'Needs assessment' for Chiswick has been broadly defined as estimating the health priorities for an individual or a population. Assessment includes both hard facts and figures as well as using the judgement of the people that work in a locality who understand the local issues and problems that occur.

It also needs to consider the demand and uptake of services. Intelligence is gathered on some of the factors that might affect demand, i.e. what other services are available in the locality, what private provision is taken up, what leisure, educational, social services and housing facilities are available and what voluntary support groups there are.

Findings. A very simple framework was developed to classify the population by age group and then used to commission services to identified needs by using care aim and health need group pairings. Table 9.3 provides an illustration of this. For each pairing, a commissioner is allowed to specify whether the service is to be offered to everyone (universal need) or if a limited number of the packages are required to meet an identified need of the local population (specified need).

Impact. Its introduction into contracting has been delayed, pending analysis of the national pilot and resolving resource issues. The anecdotal experience locally suggests that commissioners get a much clearer picture of community services and the community trust sees it as a mechanism for close monitoring of shifts of care from hospital to community.

The Horton Park Centre case study – Sandy Taylor

Objective. Bradford Community Trust and its health authority used a collaborative and participative approach to needs assessment when they wanted to develop health services in a deprived area of Bradford. This demonstrates the power of allowing a community to discuss and develop the idea which had been generated by service providers and purchasers. The central idea was the development of a 'one stop shop' delivering primary care-led health services, local authority services, voluntary sector services and a range of community facilities.

Process. The process was strongly influenced by the advice of the local authority assistant area coordinator, who provided information and ideas on the structure and composition, and the way in which the communities related to their area.

The key features of the needs assessment and service specification from the project have been:

- Involving a wide range of stakeholders – local people, local authority representatives, public health bodies, GPs, and voluntary and local organizations
- Developing and using both community intelligence and public health knowledge in determining the specification of service
- Ensuring that the area addressed makes 'sense' in community flow and use of services and facilities
- Identifying and promoting 'champions to change' to keep the energy going and to provide the impetus for the continuing development of the project.

On the advice of the assistant area coordinator, the project group agreed to start consultations with three local forums, and that it would be useful to gather names of people who would be particularly interested in forming a reference group, whose views and involvement would be sought throughout the development process.

There was a degree of anxiety within the project team about raising expectations too early and before the project funding was approved, and that they would be faced with a huge number of unrealistic, unachievable demands from these communities who may have felt they had been poorly served for some time.

Findings. However, the discussion was extremely fruitful and positive, due to the warmth of the community response to being asked for their views. There was a high degree of realism about the length of time such a

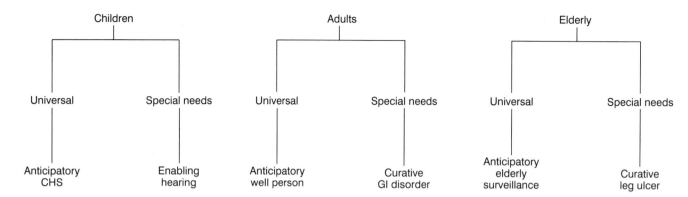

Table 9.3

project takes to come to fruition, and a clarity of thought about the priorities for health and social welfare support for their communities.

Nor were there opposing views from the different communities. The needs were, in the main, common, and specific suggestions were made about the services which the communities wanted included in the specification, including a large community space, welfare rights advice, an emphasis on women's and children's services, access to GPs out of hours as in a clinic setting, minor surgery facilities and a minor injuries clinic.

None of these suggestions might have come from a narrower view of assessing need, and the example indicated the importance of trusting communities to know what their needs are, and how they might be met, without hearing that the 'wish list' will be impossible to meet. This is perhaps of particular interest in relation to community health and primary care services, where, by and large, the needs expressed by communities are straightforward and related to improving the ability of communities to live decently, with support for their members' quality of life

Impact. At the beginning of the process there was involvement of the local GP community, with a particular focus on discovering from GPs what their feelings were about the alternative models of service being considered by the project team. These ideas were around a one stop shop with GPs located within it, or a service to which GPs would refer, but without GP presence. The project team favoured a 'GP on site' model, but were concerned that GPs in the area may have concerns about 'poaching', and thus not use the other services which would be offered by the centre. In fact, GPs thought it was important that some practices were included, which then shaped the final specification.

The final element of the needs assessment collaboration was the consultation with other front line staff from all the agencies working in the area. Staff contributed to the detailed development of the specifications, bringing their clinical knowledge and skills to the shape of the project.

Having this range of inputs into the needs assessment and service specification process has meant that the project feels well grounded in terms of being likely to meet expressed and identified need and in terms of community acceptance and ownership.

Conclusions

The role of the community trust in this needs assessment process has been as an active partner in the collaborative process – contributing knowledge and information about service need and developing the final 'blueprint', and creating access for service users and other providers into the process.

This model of needs assessment adds to the more formalized process of epidemiology and demography – and provides the qualitative 'colour' which generates a view of 'need' which is more soundly based in the community which it addresses.

The South and East Cheshire Survey of Schizophrenia – Leslie Klein

Objective. A consultant in public health from this health authority led a needs assessment involving community staff to identify:

● The numbers of people with schizophrenia
● The clinical pattern of illness
● The needs for health, social and voluntary services
● Levels of service satisfaction
● Areas of unmet need.

This work was the baseline for the service specification and subsequent tendering process for mental health services in south Cheshire.

Process. The process involved constructing an anonymized data set from agencies with contact with mental health sufferers, followed by case note review to identify schizophrenics from:

- Data from community trust community psychiatric nurses (CPNs)
- Data from social services
- Data from hospital records
- Study of GP records
- Survey of users and carers.

Findings. Some of the interesting findings included:

- One patch was under resourced, poorly managed and had poor standards of service.
- GPs had good historical and treatment data but very poor social information.
- Community trust CPNs had little idea of the historical context or contact with GPs but very accurate treatment data and social functioning data.
- Social workers (SWs) had good social data but little information on medical aspects of disease.
- There was remarkably little cross-over between CPNs and SWs, who appeared to be looking after virtually separate client groups.
- There were major disagreements about the simplest of data items (less than 30% of clients had a complete data set), CPNs saying the person was not on a Section 117 order but subject to a care programme approach, with SWs saying the reverse. People were transferred onto the care programme approach by CPNs who assumed wrongly that the Section 117 order had lapsed, and neither agency communicated with the other about subsequent management.
- Comparative to national figures a disproportionately high number of people with learning disability also suffered schizophrenia, which appeared to be due to misdiagnoses dating back to the 1950s.
- A small group of people can be identified that are very vulnerable and need moderately intensive long-term support and flexible high-dependency community services linked to an acute hospital.
- A group of about 200 people who required minimal support, but whose quality of life would substantially improve if it were provided, were identified.

Impact.

- Clinical management of some learning disabled clients was changed.
- Resource allocation was adjusted to target the under-funded patch through the relevant trust.
- Community trust management of CPNs was reviewed with proposals to:
  - Merge primary and core service that was separately controlled
  - Devise a policy which prevented swamping of CPNs with inappropriate referrals from general practice
  - Focus their skills on the vulnerable severely mentally ill
  - Devise new joint working arrangements between the community trust and the social service department, to improve coordination and recognition of priority groups.

Conclusions

Close cooperation between community trust staff, the health agency and general practice enables needs assessment to span population and individual needs, and lead to feasible service changes in both clinical practice and service pattern.

Tower Hamlets Young Rehabilitation Review – Andrew Harris

Objectives. Part of a review of services for the young physically disabled in the community trust aimed to:

1. Discern key stakeholder views on the current services, normative standards, demand, need and future service options
2. Quantitatively assess needs of population
3. Evaluate range of services
4. Make recommendations on service configuration and appropriate deployment of a consultant in rehabilitation medicine.

Process. A senior registrar in public health was attached to the trust by the regional public health training director. Part of his work involved qualitative surveys of key stakeholders. A mixture of techniques were used: a survey instrument to a critical event sample of GPs, informal conversation interviews with service heads and consumers and an open-ended survey instrument to a politically important sample of consultants. Another part involved an audit of some funded community care placements out of district, and point prevalence and annual prevalence studies of inappropriate bed occupancy due to untimely or inaccessible rehabilitation services. Epidemiological needs were assessed from analysis of census, the Office of Population Censuses and Studies (OPCS) national disability survey, the local authority disability register, specific disease prevalance rates and from selected service activity analysis.

Findings. The findings included the following:

- Services were fragmented and uncoordinated
- Information about services for users and between providers was poor
- Access to users was inequitable: Bangladeshis had greater need but lower usage of services
- Underestimates of local prevalence of non-locomotor disability on the register suggested inappropriately narrow concepts of disability

- Professional attitudes did not adequately acknowledge the social models rehabilitation
- Substantial sums were being spent on inappropriate private care out of district
- Shortages of occupational therapists and a deficiency of intermediate rehabilitation services resulted in inappropriately long stays in acute beds, especially
- 70% OT activity was plastic surgery
- Some professional staff were inadequately trained in collective goal making and planning packages of care
- A range of quality issues about waits, appointments, consultations and transport arose
- GP access to surgical appliances was demanded
- Appropriate transition from paediatric to adult care did not occur
- Changes in proposals for a local stroke unit would generate resources for establishing a comprehensive rehabilitation service in the community
- Activity and cost comparisons of an intermediate care medical ward suggested it would more appropriately be used as a mixed inpatient/day care young disabled unit.

Impact. A project officer to lead development has been appointed, and a new head of OT is refocusing service on primary care. A consultant job has been reshaped. The feasibility of the Trust acting as an agency for providing tailored packages of home care is being discussed. A joint HA/LA bid for a multidisciplinary team to oversee new rehabilitation referrals has been made, a local authority review of registration is in progress, and the DHA plan to decommission the intermediate care medical ward.

Conclusions

A service review involving assessment of perceived need

and epidemiological measures of unmet need provides the trusts with a wealth of information to address quality issues of current services and meet training and management deficits. Above all, it indicates areas where disinvestment and reshaping of services are indicated. There are market opportunities to devise new service plans as bids for continuing care are currently purchased outside the district.

The role of community health trusts in needs assessment is not to duplicate the role of commissioners, either health authority or GPs, but to ensure that their special contribution, as a multidisciplinary, multisite provider organization, bridges the gap between assessing the needs of individuals and providing care for the wider community. The diversification of public health skills into provider units is an indispensable part of this process, and should be seen as a natural development of the primary care-led NHS.

APPENDIX. ADDRESSES AND CASE STUDIES

The Chiswick Model
Julie Dent, Commissioning Director, Ealing, Hammersmith and
  Hounslow Health Agency,
  1 Armstrong Way, Southall, Middlesex UB2 4SA. Tel: 0181 967 5088

Horton Park Centre
Sandy Taylor, Chief Executive, Leeds Royal Hospital, Maudsley Street,
  Bradford BD3 9LH. Tel: 01274 363413

The South and East Cheshire Survey of Schizophrenia
Dr Leslie Klein, Consultant in Public Health, Department of Public
  Health, South and East Cheshire Health Agency, 324 Chester Road,
  Hartford, Northwich CW8 2AH. Tel: 01606 301025

Tower Hamlets Rehabilitation Review
Dr Andrew Harris, Senior Registrar in Public Health, Tower Hamlets
  Healthcare Trust, Medical Director's Office, Bancroft Unit, Mile End
  Hospital, London E1 4DG. Tel: 0717 377 7843

REFERENCES

Colin-Thomé D 1996 The Castlefields Fundholding Project
Effective Health Care Bulletin No 2 (1) 1995 The prevention and treatment of pressure sores. Effective Health Care 2 (1)
Lynch M 1995 Effect of practice and population characteristics on uptake of childhood immunisations. British Journal of General Practice 45: 205–208
Orbell S et al 1995 Assessing the effectiveness of a screening campaign: who is missed by 80% cervical screening coverage. Journal of the Royal Society of Medicine 88: 389–394

Rashid C 1995 Changing the mattress. Nursing Times 91(47)
Thomasson G 1995 Monitoring and evaluating the shift of health care services and resources from secondary to primary and community sectors. York Health Economics Consortium, York
West M, Poulton B 1995 The Micropurchasing Project. Report for Northern and Yorkshire Health Authority
Wilkinson C E et al 1992 Risk targeting in cervical screening: a new look at an old problem. British Journal of Medical Practice 42: 435–438

10

Assessing health outside the health service

David Black   *Pauline Craig*

Historically, measures of the factors affecting health were not only collected by the medical profession. The Victorian public health movement was built on data collected and decisions made by the local authority, when information was gathered on health outcomes and on social factors relating to health, such as housing, water, food quality and sewage. This wider view of the factors affecting health was lost as public health and health education became established within the health services and worked more on a medical rather than a social model of health.

Healthy public policy has its roots in this wider social definition of health. It has had a recent resurgence, supported by the World Health Organization's (WHO) policy for Health for All (HFA) and its urban development, the Healthy Cities Project. In part this has been a response to the realization of the continuing social class inequities in health, and has led to the development of a number of innovative projects tackling health issues particularly in areas of deprivation. These projects often build on the HFA principles attempting to redress inequalities in health through intersectoral collaboration and community participation, and many of them are involved in assessments of health in their local area. It is the intention of this chapter to set health needs assessment in the context of a social model of health and to describe a number of different approaches to the task, highlighting the benefits of this form of work for community health workers in the health services.

FACTORS THAT AFFECT HEALTH ARE THE RESPONSIBILITY OF US ALL

Health can be described in many ways but possibly the most common definition is that used in the constitution of the WHO:

Health is a state of complete physical, social and mental well-being and not merely the absence of disease or infirmity. The enjoyment of the highest attainable standard of health is one of the fundamental rights of every human being, without distinction of race, religion, political beliefs or economic and social conditions.   (WHO 1948)

While widely used, the important strengths of this statement are often overlooked. The first is that health is a state of being and is the outcome of a range of factors. The Lalonde Report suggested that at best health services account for only 15% of the health of the population. Most of the factors affecting health are outwith the control of the health services, therefore responsibility for the production of health in a postindustrial society is very wide and does not lie with any one organization or group. The second is that the highest attainable standard of health is a fundamental human right.

This view of health as an outcome of where you live, the resources you have and the support you receive rather than purely an artefact of your behaviour is now widely used. Sir Donald Acheson in his final report as Chief Medical Officer points out that 'The clearest links with the excess burden of ill health are: low income, unhealthy behaviour and poor housing and environmental amenities' (HMSO 1991).

As an example of the need to tackle problems on a broad front, consider the scenario of an overstretched female patient living in a damp house in a poor area, having difficulty coping on a low budget. Community health staff concerned with primary prevention, working on their own can only tackle the symptoms of this web of social issues. To address the roots of the problem they need to be part of an alliance tackling the housing, environmental, welfare benefit, employment and social policy problems of their area.

What's going on?

A collective approach to social health issues can be found in many cities and communities across the country, and assessment of health plays an important part in much of their work. In fact this is not a new movement as there has been a growing number of community-based health projects since the early 1980s. The National Community Health Resource (now Community Health UK) in its 1991 annual report pointed to information about 1500 community health initiatives in its database. Much of this work has been supported by local authority community development workers and health authority community and public health staff. Local authorities post-1974 (when they lost control over formal community/public health workers) have gradually recognized the need to be involved in a wider public health role and have developed a range of health policies and projects, most of them around the framework of the WHO Health for All philosophy. They formed a local authority health network to support this work.

This network is now part of the National Health for All Network which has 43 National Health Service (NHS) health authorities and trusts, 25 local authorities and 34 joint NHS/local authority (intersectoral) members as part of a membership of nearly 200. Part of the WHO Euronet of national networks, the UK Network is a good first port of call for contacts around the country.

The WHO interest in intersectoral action for health (Taket 1990) has provided support for a wide range of work. At national level the UK strategy documents for health (HMSO 1992, The Scottish Office 1992, Department of Health and Social Services (N Ireland), Health Promotion Wales 1990) all pay considerable attention to the role of 'healthy alliances'. The Department of Health has recently published a report on alliances in terms of the Health of the Nation (HMSO 1993). The development of the National Health for All Network as part of the European Healthy Cities Project has been a notable indicator of the wide-ranging interest in this type of work. Community involvement in local health needs assessment exercises and locality planning teams are examples of interest at a local level. Expertise in supporting and measuring this new work is being developed within the fields of public health (Funnel et al 1995) health promotion (Fieldgrass 1992) and management science (Eden & Huxham 1991) as well as within the network of projects.

WORK AT A CITY LEVEL

A number of UK cities have developed projects based on the HFA strategy. Of these, Oxford was probably the first. In 1986 they started to develop a broad health database

we were also convinced that if we were to advance health through local government we would also need to build up a general data base of health and specific data bases to validate general projects . . .. Within the Town Hall itself we bureaucrats had stored up all sorts of useful statistics from house condition surveys to gender distribution of management posts. We therefore commissioned a 'planner' to give us an inroad into this material.   (Allen 1992)

Collaborative approaches to developing descriptions of health and joint strategies to improve it can be found around the country. Work in Stockport around the Stockport Challenge is one example of health authorities and local authorities working together. The Stockport Challenge is a joint response to the health problems in the area, including those outlined in the Health of the Nation document and those missed out (e.g. poverty). It is a local health strategy which covers local authority and health authority services, targeting areas of need with enhanced services or innovative projects, and developing neighbourhood health strategies in some of these areas.

Another example is the work of the Croydon Think Tanks in addressing health inequalities in peripheral areas. These were joint pieces of work supported by Croydon Health Authority and Croydon Council to identify the causes of poor health in two peripheral areas and to propose actions to improve health. They used a combination of rapid appraisal techniques backed by public meetings and a MORI poll to check that the findings of the consultation were accurate. The final reports suggest a wide range of actions which have had a joint budget allocation of £900 000 on a recurring basis. The King's Fund suggests that: 'Joint initiatives ... should be established at the local level across the UK so that effective inter-agency strategies can be developed to tackle inequalities in health' (Benzeval et al 1995).

Many other cities have developed this approach. Health audits of local authority services, and broad-based health consultations, have been a feature of the developing work of many member projects of the Health for All Network. In this the work of the Healthy Sheffield project is worthy of note.

Glasgow – a healthy city?

The utility of collaborative approaches to health assessment can be illustrated by looking at the work of one of the four WHO pilot projects in the UK – the Glasgow Healthy City Project.

Glasgow accepted the WHO's invitation to become a member of the European Healthy Cities Pilot Project in 1988. The partner agencies in the Healthy City Project (city council, regional council, health authority, universities and voluntary sector) recognized that to tackle inequalities in health in the city they had to work together. Health had to be put back on the agenda for action at a city level, not just for individuals, or for the health authority, but for all of the organizations in the city.

The range of collaborative assessments of health which has taken place in this city using the healthy city project philosophy provides examples of the type of work which is taking place in similar situations around the country. The Glasgow project has been involved in health assessment work at all levels, some of which is listed below.

City wide

- Glasgow City Health Plan (described below)
- Glasgow Women's Health Policy (described below)
- Glasgow's Health: Women Count (described below)
- Glasgow's Health: Old Problems New Opportunities (a collaboration using already collected data to reflect new developments in the city)
- OECD Study on Health Outcomes of Housing Change

- A cohort study of children born in Glasgow (B.I.G) will make use of the wide range of collaborating partners in the project to enhance the use of its findings.

Community focused

- Kendoon Health Profile (described below)
- Concrete Action (described below)
- Dalmarnock Food and Health Study (small-area research study into access versus information in the shaping of people's food choice)
- Oatlands Health Profile (community health profile of poor areas in the south of Glasgow, used to develop support for further work)
- Easterhouse Health Needs Survey (survey commissioned by the health authority and carried out by the Council's market research team and the local Healthy City community project)
- Community health profiling exercises carried out in four areas as part of the bid for funding from Urban Aid for the Healthy City Community Support Unit (based on group interviews, discussions and the drawing together of data from a range of statutory sources)
- Perceived Health Needs of Black and Ethnic Minority Women (study carried out in the community by Healthy City Project Community Support team)
- Health Needs of the Elderly in Knightswood (health needs assessment carried out by the local community health action group with the support of the Glasgow Healthy City Project).

Topic-based work

Topic-based conferences are also used to raise the profile and information base about health issues. The Glasgow Health City Project has held two which have developed further work: Food, Poverty and Health (1992) and Gender and Health (1994).

Glasgow City Health Plan

The participating cities in the WHO European Healthy Cities Project have to produce a City Health Plan as part of their contract. These plans are collaborative in nature, and the methods used provide a good framework for health assessment at both city-wide and local levels.

Policy development

If health is an outcome of all the activities which take place in a city this means it has to have a place in the policy documents of all the cities' agencies. The Healthy City Project sought to develop this in two ways: working with the service agencies to develop a broad-based City Health Plan, and supporting the development of policy initiatives from outwith the statutory agencies.

In shaping a strategy for the development of the City Health Plan the project team decided to start with the major agencies, as it was necessary to engage their commitment if the plan was to be more than a hopeful wish list. Rooting it in the agencies allowed exploration of their perceived involvement in the health of the city and to demonstrate the implications of their work and forward plans for improving health in Glasgow.

The plan gives an overview of the city-wide work that is taking place. A model (Fig. 10.1) for the development of joint work is included, and the plans and proposals of the agencies for further work are described.

The process

Without commitment from the major decision-making forums in the city the development of the plan would have been very difficult. Access to senior management was vital in securing commitment from service departments. Representatives attended a series of intersectoral information exchanges to explore the relationships around health in the city. After a series of meetings with the participants providing written descriptions of their departments' work and relationship to health, a working document was produced.

The project team then visited all of the participants and carried out a semistructured interview exploring in more depth the plans and policy developments of the service department and their relation to health. From the results of the interviews and the draft document, a draft City Health Plan was produced.

After a period of consultation the plan was adopted by each of the three statutory agencies in the city who agreed to develop the work, ideas and issues contained in it. A joint monitoring and development group was set up to oversee implementation.

Developing the plan within the agencies took about 3 years from the start of the process to the launch of the plan. It was made possible by the strong collaborative structure and high-level commitment that the Healthy City Project had achieved over its lifetime. The launch of the document was not the end of the process but rather the beginning of the task to build even wider participation and to develop community involvement and ownership of the plan.

Monitoring, review and development

Two broad areas for further work were identified in the process. One is the need to develop a strong community input into the shaping of the plan to meet local needs. The second is to make sure that the agencies' commitments within the plan are monitored and that this work continues to be developed. It is important that the plan does not become a static document and can reflect new needs and challenges.

Women's health needs assessment

The Glasgow Healthy City Project also supports working groups to develop and bring to the attention of the city policy makers areas of health work which are under-resourced or underdeveloped. The project's Women's Health Working Group provides an example of the power of this approach. Underpinning the wide range of work which this group undertakes has been their development of a Women's Health Policy for Glasgow, now implemented by the statutory agencies. The aim of the policy is to improve the health and well-being of women in Glasgow, and it sets out recommendations to be followed whenever women's health is of concern to agencies working in the city.

This group produced a collaborative publication, *Glasgow's Health: Women Count*, a broad-based women's health needs assessment. This was the first of its kind, and has proved to be of great use in the city, and together with the policy has been used as a model for work on women's health by the WHO across Europe.

The collaborative approach to assessing health at a city-wide level is crucial. The successes of this work have given a very strong message to the project's partner organizations, providing examples for further policy developments and support for the community development work that underpins this approach.

City Health Plans have also been developed in Liverpool and Camden, and similar work has taken place in Sheffield, Oxford, Trafford, Leeds and in many of the member authorities of the HFA network.

COMMUNITY-BASED NEEDS ASSESSMENT

As part of a UK-wide survey of community action on poverty and health carried out for the Public Health Alliance (Laughlin & Black 1995), 150 poverty and health projects were investigated, many of which had carried

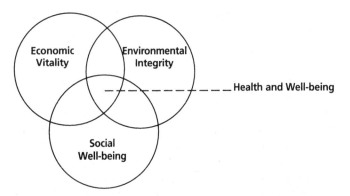

Figure 10.1 Integrated action for the creation of health (Glasgow Healthy City Project 1995; developed from an idea by T. Hancock).

out some form of health assessment. These included area-wide poverty audits which had a health component, for example, Newham Poverty Profile: Poverty on Your Doorstep, which led to the development of a multi-disciplinary health and poverty group within the council structure. It also found examples within an NHS framework, one of which, the West End Resource Centre in Newcastle, was developed with the aim of providing an effective dialogue between providers of health and social care and the local community to improve the way that the health needs of the community can be met. Local general practitioners (GPs) worked with community groups to assess the way that care can best be provided; this work led to the commissioning of a new resource centre by the health authority at a cost of £1.5 million.

There were many other projects where the local health services were working with other disciplines and with the community to get a more community focused view of health needs. In Oldham, health promotion and public health staff were involved in a local voices initiative. In Mid-Craigie in Dundee, health promotion and community health staff have supported a perceptions of health study (this was produced in two versions, traditional and cartoon). Other examples to be found in the Public Health Alliance report include the Waterfront Health Action Project, and the Glenburn Health Needs Assessment. They also note a number of health promotion departments and community nursing providers who support projects based on community development approaches, e.g. the Inequalities Initiative of the Greater Glasgow Health Board Health Promotion Department and the Stockport Health Visiting Project, both of which carry out a range of assessment exercises. The aim of the Oldham Local Voices Project sums up the nature of this type of work: 'To seek the views of local people on their health and health care needs and develop action at community and agency level to meet those needs'.

There are also a number of assessment exercises focusing on single health-related issues, e.g. food, accidents, stress and mental health. Some of these are based on community health projects, e.g. the Ferguslie Community Health Project in Strathclyde has carried out food, shopping and nutritional knowledge surveys, surveyed local children's accidents and examined stress among single parents. It used the findings to develop community-based services to address the problems they found. They have set up safety equipment loan schemes, parent support groups and a range of food, women and poverty events. Similar examples can be found in other community health projects (e.g. Pilton, Salford, etc.). In Laughlin & Black's (1995) study the two topics with most work taking place in communities were the areas of food and nutrition, and women's health.

Links between education and health services

Little work has been done in this area in Healthy Cities Projects, although examples abound of health promotion departments' local projects.

An example of a small local initiative aimed at strategically improving understanding of needs between the sectors was run by an inner London FHSA. It held a conference for school governors and heads to meet health professionals to discuss health needs. It proved a useful way of building networks and exchanging expertise on sexual health education, drugs and asthma. Health workers were surprised to learn the extent of the psychological needs of schoolchildren and the medical support and advice teachers felt they needed. It led to discussions on the role of the school nurse. The teachers were interested to have their views of asthma care challenged, and reported that the presentations would lead to different policies in schools for use of inhaled medication and attitudes to exercise (personal communication Andrew Harris).

Community health needs assessment – practice and process

Some communities have taken on large-scale health needs assessments themselves and have succeeded in bringing their priorities for health to the attention of funding organizations. Their aim is usually to gather information that they can use to negotiate improvements in services within their community.

The Kendoon Community Health Profile, Drumchapel, Glasgow

Objectives. This profile was developed to find out what residents thought about their own and their community's health, and about local health services. It used a community development process and aimed to increase local residents' participation in community health activities in general as well as gathering perceptions of health (Kennedy 1993).

Process. The epidemiological and demographic profiles of Drumchapel were noted, but the profile focused on the real-life experience of health and illness of around 100 Drumchapel residents and their families. The profile group who planned and executed the process comprised seven local residents and seven workers from the Glasgow Healthy City Project, health promotion, health visiting, the local volunteer centre, community work, housing and an addictions project. Data were gathered by structured interviews with residents of Kendoon Avenue, and had a response rate of 97%. The questionnaire was written by the profile group based on issues prioritized from 'brainstorming' sessions at a series of open meetings.

Findings. The main health issues that were identified as being most important to Drumchapel residents included:

- The need for a new health centre, with health information and counselling services, a patient/user's group and a crèche
- More local support for people experiencing emotional difficulties such as self-help groups and individual counselling
- The threat that traffic posed to children, with lack of play areas and childcare facilities
- Damp housing and the depressing and hazardous nature of the local surroundings
- A need for self-help and discussion groups on a range of women's health issues.

In common with most community development work, some of the outcomes were not predicted.

Impact. The group produced a report and video which have been used as negotiating tools for raising awareness of issues in funding organizations and for training other community groups in needs assessment. The health profile identified the need for a coordinated approach to community health activity and laid the groundwork for the development of a project now known as Drumming Up Health (Drumchapel Community Health Project). Some of the profile group members went on to form the core groups in this project: its community health volunteer scheme and its working group. A health promotion officer from the Greater Glasgow Health Board and a health visitor from the Community and Mental Health Trust were seconded to develop the project along with two workers employed directly by the project. The community health volunteers and staff worked together to develop a number of community-led initiatives including a network of self-help and support groups, local health forums, a community health magazine and a men's health project.

Drumming Up Health continues to use the community health profile model as a framework for ongoing health needs assessment and prioritizing of issues for development. For example, the community health volunteers took on the issue of children's play areas. They researched the topic in more depth by doing a postal survey of parents of primary and nursery school children and assessing the condition of existing play areas in Drumchapel. A report was produced (Concrete Action) with recommendations that were taken on board by a number of local policy-making bodies, including the Parks and Recreation Department of Glasgow District Council. The play area research also gave rise to a group that campaigned successfully for the building of a new showpiece safe play area, and a loan scheme for home safety equipment.

The need for counselling services identified by the Kendoon Community Health Profile, together with a growing interest in complementary therapies by community health volunteers and other project users, led to an off-shoot project called One-to-One. Counselling, aromatherapy and shiatsu are offered free of charge to Drumchapel residents and are complemented by a Tai Chi class set up by Drumming Up Health. The health visitor based at Drumming Up Health took on the role of gatekeeper at One-to-One, offering an initial consultation with potential clients and referring on either to the One-to-One therapists or to other statutory or voluntary agencies. Clients came initially from the community health volunteers, the support groups and by 'word-of-mouth', but after 2 years more than two-thirds of referrals came from Drumchapel GPs. It appears that 5 years after the community health profile, GPs began to recognize a need among their patients for counselling and self-help.

Community Needs Project, Stewartstown, Near Belfast

This project, coordinated by a health visitor and funded by Making Belfast Work, worked with the local population to help identify health needs, survey those needs and work in various ways to lobby and campaign for the issues identified to be tackled and improved. It was funded for 3 years and based around two housing schemes between Lisburn and Belfast.

Process. The project was over a 3 year time period, and the process was as follows:

1. Establishing a management team (Making Belfast Work management and community health services management)
2. Establishing links with the community and local representative committee was aided by the coordinator having worked in the area for the past 12 years
3. Unstructured focus groups exploring categories of service to be developed and changed, e.g. new services, services to be continued and services to be removed
4. Pilot survey to prepare an interview schedule involving local groups and representatives
5. Random sample of population prepared
6. 625 interviews of householders and young people carried out by trained local volunteer interviewers
7. Parallel interviews of fieldworkers' (teachers, youth club leaders, health service staff, etc.) perceptions of local needs for comparative purposes
8. Coding of questionnaires
9. Production of a report based on qualitative data, i.e. focus groups
10. Discussion with community groups

11. Writing up the main report
12. Local people and project coordinator working together to report back findings to the community, discuss how the findings can be used and plan strategies for taking up key issues.

It should not be thought beyond the role and responsibilities of general practices to escape in this type of assessment. What is needed is an understanding of its value and an attitude to be keen to listen to and exchange with others, experiences of work in the same community. It makes routine general practice work more fulfilling, and developing the networks creates opportunities and opens doors that were previously closed. It also enables other professionals to understand better the pressures, demands and role of GPs. Two examples, one on a very small scale, without funding, show unpredictable benefits.

The Camberley Surgery Project

Objective. The aim was to explore interagency concerns which influenced service need and develop a health profile.

Process. The project established a group with a representative of the users, FHSA, community trust, acute trust, midwifes, voluntary services, environmental health, housing, social services and police.

Findings. It was found that data collected by most organizations was inappropriate to the needs profile and based on different areas, and there was a higher than average accident and emergency department attendance rate.

Impact. The impact was threefold:

● The police began to collect data on domestic violence and drugs on geographic ward basis
● A multiagency group was established to facilitate command and useful data collection and exchange between organizations
● Social services allocated a practice-attached social worker.

Wells Park Health Project

Process. The Wells Park Health Project (B. Fisher, personal communication) is a community development organization working closely with the Wells Park general practice. Since 1991, the FHSA has been supporting the project almost completely, funding two full-time community workers, one administrative worker and one part-time community work student. It is managed by a committee of local people and professionals, including a nurse and a GP from the practice. Founded on community development principles, the project believes that by bringing people together, usually in groups, support can

be given and empowerment can begin. Networking and support links are regarded as important in improving health.

Objectives.

● To provide services within the project's capacity in response to local need
● To develop needs assessment from a lay point of view with an emphasis on ethnic minority work
● To develop methodology that will fuse the qualitative, action-oriented community development with a quantitative research base
● To find a way to use the information gained to influence purchasing decisions of the health commission
● To continue to involve local people in determining the direction of the project.

Impact. Needs assessment has focused on population groups such as young people, the Afro-Caribbean community and the elderly housebound and their carers. Outcomes of the project have included the development of several groups, a health library and a housing forum.

The project has also stimulated a number of changes within local health service provision:

● General practice opening times and appointment system
● Free acupuncture and osteopathy service
● Changes in cervical cytology procedures
● New bus service in hilly area
● Health authority funding proposals for a youth health worker and community development mental health worker for the Afro-Caribbean community
● Proposal for new Department of Health recommendations for opticians and dentists, calling up young people directly (from the youth health needs assessment).

LINKS WITH COMMUNITY HEALTH WORKERS

Many community-based health needs assessments are carried out by health service workers in collaboration with their communities using community development approaches. For example, in Liverpool two health visitors were employed as public health nurses to facilitate the compilation of locality profiles (D. Colin-Thomé, personal communication). Their aim was to raise awareness within the primary care team of the public health needs of their local population and for the team to recognize the role they could play in the health of their community as a whole, not only for their practice lists. They believed that for primary care teams to provide primary prevention they must understand the needs of the population they serve. A community development approach enabled a number of community initiatives to be developed from the general practice (Cernik & Wearne 1992). A similar approach was taken in Edinburgh by a primary care team, and is discussed elsewhere in this book. They also recognized the benefits of primary care as a setting for assessing wider public health and health service needs of both patients and communities (Murray 1995).

Finally in Stockport, five whole time equivalent (wte) health visiting posts were created to work in deprived areas with a remit to work with groups to facilitate identification of the communities' own health needs and to develop communal ways of addressing the needs. Initiatives implemented in the communities include an Asian women's exercise group, a credit union and a food cooperative. The scheme has also been instrumental in stimulating changes in the health visiting service across Stockport, which has become more consumer focused (Smith 1995). The Strelley Nursing Development Unit also supported a public health/community development model for their health visitors, who were able to facilitate the setting up of a range of community groups and services (Boyd et al 1993).

CONCLUSION

There has been a marked growth in the numbers of community health projects over the last 15 years. Some support has come from the health services for the projects in confronting the complex web of issues that shape health and ill-health in our society. There certainly is evidence that methods used within community health projects have stimulated health services in some areas into incorporating a more realistic appraisal of health needs into their own processes. Along with recognition of the complexity of the concept of 'health', there is the realization that health needs assessment must reflect people's lives as well as national mortality figures.

The scientific community may regard the methods described as worthy responses to expressed need, or demand, but not strictly needs assessment. But where there is strong triangulation across groups (see Ch. 2) it is legitimate to describe those methods as assessments, reflecting population needs, due to the consensus achieved. This is supplemented by Ong et al (1991), who described a triangulation with informants from those groups with knowledge of the community, gained through their help within community groups, e.g. voluntary workers, those who had that knowledge through their profession, e.g. social workers, and those who were centrally placed because of their role in the community, e.g. turf accountants (Ong et al 1991). The weakness in their case is that the interviewees were exposed to so many common influences (e.g. media, some health services, socio-economic status, etc.) that it cannot be said that they formed their perspectives from independent sources. Nevertheless, it gives a normative balance to expressed need, and should be included in overall needs assessment processes.

The community health project work links medical and social models of health, allowing GPs and other health care workers access to networks within their communities addressing the structural factors affecting health, e.g. housing, transport and food access. These approaches are not sterile technical solutions to health needs assessment but, hopefully, the start of local collaborative work leading to Health For All.

We hope that this chapter has given a taster of some of the collaborative work on health that is taking place around the country. That this work is important and developing can be seen in a number of recent publications and reports; but a better indication of the richness of the work and its outcomes can be found in speaking to some of the participants and workers in these types of projects. Appendix 2 gives some contact points to help you get in touch with local projects.

APPENDIX 1. ORGANIZATIONS AND NETWORKS FOCUSED ON HEALTH/COMMUNITY DEVELOPMENT

National Food Alliance London, 3rd Floor, 5/11 Worship Street, London EC2A 2BH. Tel.: 0171 628 2442

Health for All Network, PO Box 101, Liverpool L69 5BE

Health Visitors' Association, 50 Southwark Street, London SE1 1UN. Tel.: 0171 378 7255

UK Health for All Network, PO Box 101, Liverpool L69 5BE. Tel.: 0151 231 1009

Public Health Alliance, 138 Digbeth, Birmingham B5 6DR. Tel.: 0121 643 7628

Royal College of Nursing (Public Health Nursing Group), 20 Cavendish Square, London W1M 0AB. Tel.: 0171 409 3333

Community Health UK (used to be the National Community Health Resource Unit), 6 Terrace Walk, Bath BA1 1LN. Tel.: 01225 464 680

Community Health Development Adviser, Save The Children Fund UK, 6 Western Corner, Edinburgh EH12 5PY. Tel.: 0131 346 8352

APPENDIX 2. ADDRESSES OF PROJECTS

Camberley Surgery Project
Drs Geoff Roberts and Liz Anstead,
    Upper Gordon Road Surgery, Camberley, Surrey, GU15 2HJ

Community Development Health Promotion Officer – Dundee
Sylvia Somerville,
    Tayside Health Promotion Centre, 7 Dudhope Terrace, Dundee DD3 6HG. Tel.: 01382 228213
Aims/objectives:
    To support and develop health related initiatives at community level using community development

Glenburn Health Project
John Thomson,
    St Peters Primary School, Braehead Road, Paisley PA2 8DZ. Tel.: 0141 884 8542
Aims/objectives:
    1. Promote and establish a health forum for the Glenburn area composed of local residents, activists and professionals who work in the area
    2. Promote the health of the Glenburn community in a proactive manner – do this in conjunction with a health needs assessment and locally perceived needs

Ferguslie Community Health Project
Bill Grey,
    The Tannahill Centre, Ferguslie Park, Paisley. Tel.: 0141 887 9650
Aims/objectives:
    The project adopts a non-pathological non-victim-blaming
    philosophy along with a community development practice in an
    attempt to encourage and enable local groups and individuals to
    better understand and where appropriate tackle the factors affecting
    the health of themselves, their families and their community

Healthy Sheffield
Liz Gaere,
    Westbrook House, Sharrowvale Road, Sheffield S11 8EV. Tel.: 0114
    273 4645
Aims/objectives:
    To promote the health and well being of the people of Sheffield by
    addressing a wide range of environmental, economic and social issues

Inequalities Initiative, GGHB
Trevor Lakey,
    Health Promotion Department, 225 Bath Street, Glasgow G2 4JT.
    Tel.: 0141 201 4444
Aims/objectives:
    Piloting methods and approaches to promoting the health of people
    in disadvantaged groups as a contribution to the long-term goal of
    reducing inequalities in health

London Borough of Newham Anti-poverty Strategy; Health and Poverty Work
Rita Davies,
    3 Nelson Street, East Ham, London E6 4EQ. Tel.: 0181 472 1430 x23878
Aims/objectives:
    To address health and poverty issues identified in the Newham
    poverty profile 'Poverty on your doorstep'

Oldham Local Voices Initiative
Diane Charlesworth,
    Health Promotion Department, West Pennine Health Authority,
    Westhulme Avenue, Oldham 0LI 2PL. Tel.: 0161 455 5750
Aims/objectives:
    To seek the views of local people on their health and health care
    needs and develop action at community and agency levels to meet
    those needs

Pilton Health Project
Kate Burton,
    The Health Hut, 3 West Pilton Park, Edinburgh EH4 4EL. Tel.: 0131
    332 0871
Aims/objectives:
    To use a community development approach in encouraging
    awareness and action on health issues in the area

Stewartstown Community Needs Project
Barbara Murphy,
    Stewartson Road Health Centre, Stewartson Road, Dunmurry,
    Belfast BT17 0FB. Tel.: 01232 602931
Aims/objectives:
    To work with the population of a disadvantaged area in order to
    help them to identify their health needs, survey these needs and
    work in various ways to pressurize/campaign for the issues
    identified to be changed/improved

Salford Community Health Project
Karen McCarthy,
    Higher Broughton Health Centre, Bevenden Square, Salford M7
    0UF. Tel.: 0161 792 6969
Aims/objectives:
    This project aims to listen to what people say and is important for a
    healthy life. It aims to: help people get their voices heard so that
    services can be more suited to their communities; help people get
    together and meet others to offer support, understanding and
    information; work with other workers locally and across Salford, to
    try and influence decisions which affect people's health

Stockport Community Health Worker Projects
Joan Fletcher,
    Brinnington Health Centre, Brinnington Road, Brinnington,
    Stockport. Tel.: 0161 430 3383
Aims/objectives:
    To adopt a holistic approach to health by facilitating individual and
    collective action around the felt needs of the community

West End Health Resource Centre
Dr Chris Drinkwater,
    Department of Primary Health Care, The Medical School,
    Framlington Place, Newcastle upon Tyne NE2 4HH. Tel.: 0191 222
    8769
Aims/objectives:
    To provide a focus for an effective dialogue between providers of
    health and social care and the local community about the ways in
    which their health needs should be met, both in terms of
    preventative strategies and service delivery

Wells Green Community Health Project
Dr B. Fisher,
    The Wells Park Practice, 1 Wells Park Road, London SE26

Waterfront Health Action Project
David Wainright,
    221 Erith Road, Bexleyheath, Kent. Tel.: 0181 302 2678 x2568
Aims/objectives:
    The improvement in health and well-being of people in the
    waterfront area through partnership between local residents and
    health and welfare professionals

Glasgow Healthy City Project
Glasgow City Council,
    227 George Street, Glasgow G2 1DU Tel.: 0141 287 4317
Aims/objectives:
    To make Glasgow a healthier city through joint work by
    community, statutory and voluntary agencies. To develop and
    implement the City Health Plan. To reduce health inequalities

Drumming Up Health
Drumchapel Health Centre,
    80–90 Kinfauns Drive, Glasgow G15 7TX. Tel.: 0141 211 6166
Aims/objectives:
    To coordinate, resource and support community health activity in
    line with HFA principles. To develop mechanisms to address health
    inequalities. To help residents take control of their health

REFERENCES

Allen P 1992 Off the rocking horse; how local councils can promote your health and environment. Green Print / Merlin

Avan G 1995 Perceived health needs of black and ethnic minority women. Glasgow Healthy City Project, Glasgow

Benzeval M, Judge K, Whitehead M 1995 Tackling inequalities in health: an agenda for action. King's Fund, London

Black D, Womersley J (ed) 1993 Glasgow's health: old problems new opportunities. Greater Glasgow Health Board, Glasgow

Boyd M, Brummell K, Billingham K, Perkins E 1993 The public health post at Strelley; an interim report. Nottingham Community Health NHS Trust, Nottingham

Cernik K, Wearne M 1992 Using community health profiles to improve service provision. Health Visitor 65(10): 343–345

Craig P A 1995 A different role: health visiting in a community project. Glasgow Healthy City Project, Glasgow

Department of Health and Social Services, N Ireland 1993 Regional strategy for the N Ireland health and personal social services

Draper P 1991 Health through public policy; the greening of public health. Green Print / Merlin

Drumchapel Community Health Project. 1992 Concrete action (for Drumchapel docs)

Eden C, Huxham C 1991 Tackling social issues through inter-organisational collaboration: development of a methodology for evaluating and redesigning the collaborative process. Department of Management Science, Strathclyde University, Strathclyde

Fieldgrass J 1992 Partnerships in health promotion: collaboration between the statutory and voluntary sectors. HEA / NCVO

Funnel R, Oldfield K, Speller V 1995 Towards healthier alliances. HEA and Wessex Institute of Public Health

Glasgow Healthy City Project 1995 Glasgow City Health Plan (for GHCP docs)

Hair S 1994 Glasgow's health: women count. Glasgow Healthy City Project, Glasgow

Health Promotion Wales 1990 Health for all in Wales.

HMSO 1991 Chief Medical Officer: on the state of the public health 1990. HMSO, London

HMSO 1992 The health of the nation. HMSO, London

HMSO 1993 Working together for better health, the health of the Nation. HMSO, London

Kennedy A 1993 Local voices – local lives: the story of the Kendoon Community Health Profile. Drumchapel Community Health Project, Drumchapel

Laughlin S, Black D 1995 Poverty and health: tools for change. Public Health Alliance, Birmingham.

Murray S 1995 Practice based health needs assessment: use of four methods in a small neighbourhood. British Medical Journal 310: 1443–1448

National Food Alliance 1994 Food and low income. A practical guide for advisors and supporters working with families and young people on low income. National Food Alliance, London

Ong B N, Humphris G, Annett H, Rifkin S 1991 Rapid appraisal in an urban setting, an example from the developed world. Social Science and Medicine 32(8): 909–915

Smith J 1995 The Stockport experience in visions for the future. HVA, London

Taket A R (ed) 1990 Making partners: intersectoral action for health. World Health Organization, Geneva

The Scottish Office 1992 Scotland's Health. A challenge to us all

UK Health for All Network 1993 Health for All Starter Pack. UK Health for All Network, Liverpool

WHO 1948 WHO constitution. World Health Organization, Geneva

11

Community assessment techniques for general practices

Scott A. Murray   Stephen Gillam

General practitioners and community nurses observe patients' health over long periods of time and in the context of families and communities. Primary care is thus an appropriate setting for describing the wider public health and health service needs of both patients and communities. Previous chapters have shown how practical and valid methods of assessing the needs of practice populations or the residents of specific neighbourhoods can inform the provision of primary and secondary care. This chapter tries to bring these together. It presents three overlapping approaches to needs assessment in primary care. A theme emphasized in Chapter 2 was the prerequisite for productive needs assessment: a shared view within the practice of its importance. This orientation cannot be taken for granted. The community-oriented primary care approach is one solution to the problem of integrating management and needs assessment discussed in relation to localities in Chapter 8, as it places profiling activities in the planning context.

Busy primary health care teams (PHCTs) need practical models and the following sections describe different approaches used in one urban practice. Of these methods, rapid appraisal, which addressed the wider health problems raised in Chapter 10, by directly involving community representatives, proved most successful in effecting change. The final section on community profiling shows how some of the techniques discussed in earlier chapters can be combined to improve effectiveness of assessment, in a general practice setting.

COMMUNITY-ORIENTED PRIMARY CARE
Introduction

Community-oriented primary care (COPC) is the continual process by which PHCTs provide care to a defined community on the basis of its assessed health needs by the planned integration of public health with primary care practice (King's Fund 1994). It is based on a set of principles that have been operationalized in different ways in different places and stands in a long tradition of attempts to fuse the practice of public health medicine and primary medical care (Toon 1994).

The principles of COPC were first formally delineated by Sydney Kark (1974, 1981). His ideas grew out of the experience of attempting to provide appropriate services in deprived areas of rural South Africa. They were refined following his subsequent emigration to Israel. The conceptual basis of COPC can be identified in the writings of Will Pickles (1939), but Julian Tudor-Hart's studies of hypertension from Glyncorryg provide the most notable British examples of COPC (Hart 1988).

The importance of public health skills in general practice is recognized increasingly, and COPC may offer an appropriate methodology for helping develop them. The King's Fund COPC package includes educational materials for use in structured workshops with practice-based teams and health service managers (Gillam et al 1994).

Process – The COPC cycle (Fig. 11.1)

An assessment of the practice population's health needs is carried out in three stages. For the *community diagnosis* the PHCT defines the health problems of their community on the basis of available quantitative and qualitative data (Table 11.1). This includes team members' local knowledge derived from working in the community over years. Each PHCT produces a comprehensive list of the major health-related problems in their practice population (Box 11.1).

The second stage is *prioritization*. A simple grid is used to score each health problem in relation to specific criteria, e.g. size of the problem, availability of an effective intervention, acceptability to the team and the consumer, feasibility, community involvement and resource requirements (Fig. 11.2).

Having selected one health problem, the teams next explore the extent of the priority problem in the total

Table 11.1 Data used for community diagnosis in COPC[a]

Source	Examples
Practice environment	Physical location, topographical features, transport, physical description of surgery premises, local employment, housing, local environmental risk factors
Community characteristics	Practice list age/sex breakdown, socioeconomic status, ethnic minorities (numbers and special needs), deprivation indices, unemployment rates
State of health Morbidity	Data on patients with chronic diseases (e.g. hypertension, heart failure, stroke, asthma, diabetes), antenatal and births data, teenage conception rates, termination rates, infectious disease notifications, specialist referral rates, inpatient admission rates
Mortality	Local ward level standardized mortality ratios specific (e.g. congenital heart disease, lung cancer)
Risk factors	Behavioural data on smoking, alcohol consumption, dietary, exercise patterns, substance misuse, sexual behaviour
Health service system Within the practice	Number of general practitioners, nurses, other practice-attached staff, special interests, complementary therapy, patient turnover rate
Outside the practice	Health services (e.g. hospital and community) and voluntary services (e.g. meals on wheels) gap analysis

[a] Much data on this list will tend to be available at ward not practice level. Care is required in its interpretation.

practice population – the *detailed assessment*. This constitutes a baseline for later evaluation. The inclusion of non-users is a cardinal feature of COPC. The teams use their own and local expert knowledge as well as specialist literature.

Intervention plans should define relevant activities, who is responsible for their implementation, records required, training needs, milestones and deadlines. Realistic objectives must be clearly defined. District health authorities (DHAs) and family health service authorities (FHSAs) have provided limited extra resources and advice for survey design, questionnaire development, data processing and analysis.

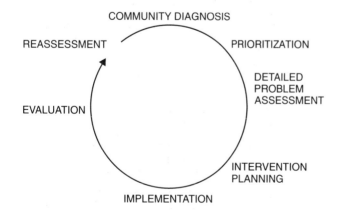

Figure 11.1 The COPC cycle.

COMMUNITY DIAGNOSIS
REASSESSMENT
PRIORITIZATION
DETAILED PROBLEM ASSESSMENT
EVALUATION
INTERVENTION PLANNING
IMPLEMENTATION

Box 11.1 A selection of typical COPC project topics

- Smoking
- Cardiovascular risk factors in middle age
- Urinary incontinence
- Health behaviours in adolescence
- Depression in women
- School health
- People taking minor tranquillizers
- Hypertension in ethnic minorities
- Sexual health in young people
- Anxiety and depression among Tamils

CRITERION	HEALTH PROBLEMS					
	Coughs and colds	Postnatal depression	Carers	Asthma	Smoking	Cancer
Prevalence/incidence	3	3	3	3	3	3
Severity of problems	1	3	3	3	3	3
Effective intervention	1	3	3	3	2	1
Acceptability/feasibility	1	3	2	2	3	2
Community involvement	1	2	3	2	2	2
Costs and resources	3	2	2	2	2	2
TOTAL SCORE	10	16	16	15	15	13

Figure 11.2 An example of a prioritization grid.

The teams then consider the methods they will use to assess the degree to which programme objectives have been met. Early definition of the data required for the *evaluation* is a critical part of the COPC process.

In the final *reassessment* phase, a decision is made as to whether or not to continue the particular intervention in the light of the evaluation. The community diagnosis is revisited prior to re-entering the COPC cycle.

The King's Fund COPC pilot programme

The King's Fund initiated a COPC pilot programme in Northumberland in 1991. Eight practices from three further sites (Sheffield, Winchester and Haringey (in north London)) joined the programme in 1992. Pilot practices received local support from their FHSA and DHA. The King's Fund funded the initial workshops and additional support in the form of process consultancy. An evaluation of the King's Fund programme focused on three areas: the impact of the COPC on the teams, its impact on patients, and cost-effectiveness.

Findings

The pilot project yielded quantifiable benefits for patients. Unlike much locality needs assessment, it appears that needs were translated rapidly into services, perhaps because it was part of the planning cycle, at the practice level. Patient-related outcomes of the 11 COPC projects are summarized in Table 11.2. In the practices focusing on coronary heart disease, these amounted to increases in risk factor coverage and the identification of new smokers, people with hypertension and raised serum cholesterol levels.

Impact

The impact of COPC projects is summarized in Table 11.3.

Participation in the COPC project helped to develop skills in protocol development, needs assessment, project management, monitoring and evaluation. The two cases studies (Boxes 11.2 and 11.3) illustrate the potential

Table 11.2 Summary of patient-related outcomes in COPC projects

Practice	Outcomes
1	Increased coverage of cardiovascular risk factors in age group 25–74 years by 950 (21%). Newly identified smokers (223) and hypertensives (81). Stop smoking clinic established
2	Increased coverage of cardiovascular risk factors (247 screened). Newly identified smokers (58), hypertensives (38), patients with raised serum cholesterol (88 borderline, 28 high) and heavy drinkers (15)
3	Trained 14 community counsellors. Counselling/advice given to more than 100 patients
4	Newly identified smokers (127), cessation documented in 17. Stop smoking clinic and individual counselling for smokers established
5	1331 patients newly screened. Newly identified smokers (348), hypertensives (31) and moderate/heavy drinkers (166)
6	Practice-based continence service established, 47 women treated
7	264 people screened. Patients with risk factors newly identified (127)
8	779 (70.6%) patients aged between 40 and 50 years surveyed regarding smoking habits with follow-up at 1 year. Cessation documented in 31
9	Recorded screening coverage increased by 851 (28.5%) for males and 933 (42.3%) for females aged 40–64 years
10	80 (31% of those invited) patients screened on 40th birthday and 74 (40%) on their 50th birthday
11	51 new patients with asthma identified via postal questionnaire and telephone survey. 483 patients' blood pressure newly measured. New services for bereaved, mother and toddlers, elderly, adolescents

Table 11.3 Summary of the impact of COPC projects

Impact of COPC on the PHCT	Impact of COPC on patient services in five practices
Helped develop participant skills	Stop smoking clinic established
Increased mutual understanding	14 new community counsellors trained and services expanded
Learnt theoretical limitations to data	Smoker's counselling service established
Gained motivation through greater sense of autonomy	Bereavement, mother and toddler, elderly and adolescent services begun

role of the COPC process in defining hitherto 'neglected' health problems in a community. However, this work is time-consuming. Assessment of health needs at practice level requires the collation of various sources of data. The intimate knowledge of a neighbourhood derived from years at the coal-face is easily undervalued as 'anecdotal' or 'qualitative'. Often, it cannot be bettered. The contribution of community nursing staff is particularly important. COPC appeared to increase mutual understanding among participants.

The state of development of practice information systems was an important factor affecting the momentum of the project. The discipline of focused data collection, analysis and evaluation developed computer literacy among key individuals. Relating ward-based census data to practice populations is difficult, particularly in urban areas. The PHCTs were inclined to jump to superficial conclusions when care was not taken to explain the theoretical limitations of data. The small size of practice populations determined that statistically significant changes in most outcome measures were unlikely to be detected for any but common conditions.

Health of the Nation priorities may not be equally relevant to all practice populations. Ownership is critical for the successful undertaking of new areas of pre-

---

Box 11.2 COPC case study 1

A rural practice initially ranked cardiovascular disease as their highest priority. However, the team felt that they were already investing a great deal of effort in this area. In discussing other priorities a practice nurse drew attention to a major cause of distress to affected patients: urinary incontinence. The doctors initially did not appreciate the extent of the problem. In the words of the nurse: 'You don't see it. We're always replacing the leaflets on incontinence. They come to us.' The team elected to accept this as their priority. A prevalence study has been performed on women aged 40–49 years with a 75% response rate. The results show that only 31% have never had an episode of incontinence and that 23% could be defined as having marked incontinence. The intervention included both preventive exercises, community education and the setting up of a local continence clinic by a specially trained practice nurse.

Box 11.3 COPC case study 2

A fundholding urban practice has used the COPC process imaginatively. Beginning with a single project on hypertension, the team has moved on to identify a range of subjects for investigation and intervention. This now includes people with asthma, elderly people with special needs, mothers with young babies and the bereaved. The presentation of an individual clinical case problem at a practice meeting elicits the question: what is the extent of the problem in the community as a whole? All staff are involved in the decision-making process.

---

ventive work in general practice. Many general practitioners feel 'over-managed'. The sense of greater autonomy that COPC provided was in itself motivating for PHCTs.

What distinguishes COPC from most practice-based audits is its starting point. Traditionally, in selecting audit topics, doctors have begun with concerns of their own. COPC uses a more objective community profiling exercise against which to select priorities. The pilot project has demonstrated that COPC can offer a useful framework for fundholding practices seeking to develop needs-led purchasing plans. The principles of COPC may also be relevant to the development of locality purchasing where systematic approaches to the assessment of small areas' health needs are often lacking.

In five practices, new services were established. These have been sustained thus far. The long-term impact of the practice-based continence service and community counselling is difficult to assess. For those practices where information was available, COPC appeared cost-effective. Preventive interventions are highly cost-effective, and stopping only for smoking offset the average costs of a COPC project.

Conclusions

A commitment to improve the whole practice population's health requires an understanding of those patients not in regular contact with the practice. COPC enables PHCTs to adopt a more systematic and rigorous approach to community health needs assessment, prioritization of local health problems, and the identification of effective health interventions based on sound research. PHCTs who can apply public health frameworks to their work will better understand the commissioning process.

COPC is best seen as an inclusive set of general principles providing the basis for the development of new forms of joint learning. COPC does not provide a radically new way of delivering health services in the UK setting. It should be used to complement other initiatives that aim to increase understanding of the factors influencing the health of practice populations and how to address them.

RAPID PARTICIPATORY APPRAISAL

Introduction

Rapid participatory appraisal, initially pioneered in the field of agricultural development in developing countries, is a qualitative technique for community assessment which can yield valuable insights into a community's own perspectives of its needs. In Britain, Ong et al in 1991 used this action research method to define health and social needs in a large urban deprived community. Its use was recognized as a means to involve local people in planning and monitoring health interventions, as well as a means by which to develop and maintain intersectoral and multidisciplinary planning. Cresswell in 1992 utilized this method in a smaller population in Derbyshire. This method is being increasingly used throughout the UK.

The general framework of rapid appraisal is based on the Health for All 2000 philosophy of equity, participation, and a multisectoral approach. The team conducting the investigations is derived from various organizations and not just health workers. The attitudes and skills necessary include a willingness to learn from local people, careful listening during interviews and informal conversations, awareness and sensitivity to everything that can be directly observed, and the use of common sense in analysing the information. A willingness to reinterpret hypotheses as information is available is vital.

The primary aims of rapid appraisal are:

1. To gain insight into a community's own perspective on its priority needs
2. To translate these findings into action
3. To establish an ongoing relationship between service purchasers, providers and local communities.

Process

Rapid appraisal may involve collecting information on nine areas of activity in four layers. The conceptual framework of the information pyramid is shown in Figure 11.3. The bottom layer defines the composition of the community, how it is organized, and its capacities to act. The second layer covers the socioecological factors which influence health. The next layer covers data on the existence, coverage, accessibility and acceptability of services, which allows an evaluation of the effectiveness of present provision, and provides a method of assessing what could usefully be changed. The final level is concerned with national, regional and local policies. The pyramid shape is a reminder that in this method success depends on building a planning process which rests on a strong community information base.

Data are collected from three main sources:

1. Existing written records about the neighbourhood
2. Interviews with a range of informants

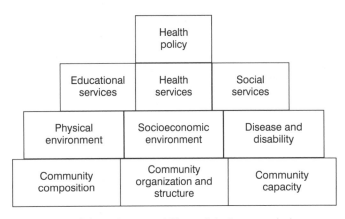

Figure 11.3   Information pyramid for participatory appraisal.

3. Observations made in the neighbourhood or in the homes of interviewees.

From the information thus collected the 'pyramid' describing the problems, priorities, and potential solutions of the neighbourhood can be drafted.

The scientific rigour and validity of this approach depends on the concept of triangulation, with data collection from one source being validated or rejected by checking it with data from at least two other sources or methods of collection. Through cross-checking observations among divergent data sources, apparent differences may resolve themselves and a favoured coherent interpretation may be constructed (Brody 1992). Informants are not selected randomly, but 'purposefully' or strategically (Johnson 1990). Thus the people who are thought to be in the best position to understand the issues are asked. Confirming and disconfirming opinions are sought. Manderson & Aaby (1992) have reviewed issues relating to the representativeness, reliability and validity of these rapid methods. The *Rapid Rural Appraisal Notes* series shares current experiences and methods among practitioners of these methods throughout the world. A special issue on applications for health was published (Welbourne 1992).

Case study – application of participatory appraisal (Murray et al 1994, Murray 1995)

Dumbiedykes, a small council estate of 670 homes in central Edinburgh, was studied. It contains a relatively homogeneous community, and half of the residents were patients of Mackenzie Medical Centre. The health visitor attached to that practice, the local community education worker, and two local social workers were brought together by a general practitioner who wished to foster a community development approach. As the team could not work full time on the project, the study was done over 3 months, with team members giving about 4 hours each week to the project. A part-time secretary was recruited for this period.

The research team devised a semistructured interview schedule (see Appendix 1) which was refined during pilot interviews. The interview training material available from the World Health Organization was useful, and has since been updated (World Health Organization 1995). The key informants were identified from various backgrounds (see Appendix 2). They included people with professional knowledge about the community, community leaders of self-help groups and voluntary organizations, and people who were centrally placed because of their work. Also, 17 residents were selected to represent various age groups, social situations, and health problems. Several group interviews were carried out. During some interviews new informants emerged, and these people were also interviewed. Participants were visited by two team members in their homes or at work. One interviewer talked to the respondent and the other took notes. The doctor and health visitor did not interview together in case such interviews would concentrate too narrowly on a medical definition of health.

Data from written documents, interviews, and observations were allotted to appropriate blocks of the planning pyramid by opening a box file for each block. Data from each interview were split into the 10 separate areas and allocated to each file. The data from all interviews were collated with other sources of information such as the 1991 census.

A feedback meeting was held to present the findings to all informants. After this, two focus groups were set up to discuss and allot priority to the problems identified and to explore potential interventions. These groups also discussed how to improve the uptake of existing services and suggested new ways to meet gaps in services. Two researchers sat in each group to facilitate and record the findings. A report was circulated by the research team, and the local newspaper reported the study in detail and invited comments on the findings and proposals.

Findings

Some of the findings are shown in Box 11.4, demonstrating Dumbiedykes' residents considered that poor transport, dog fouling, poverty, drug abuse and lack of information about services impacted on their health.

Impact

Due to the interactive nature of this action research method, a number of improvements in services had

---

Box 11.4 Some findings of the Dumbiedykes study

Community composition
- Many elderly (twice the number in the 1974 census)
- Newcomers frequently had medical or social problems
- Few children
- Little opportunity to meet except in lifts or waiting for a bus

Community organizations and capacity for change
- Very few services in Dumbiedykes
- Community Centre not known to everyone
- Three church house groups

Physical environment
- Hills and difficult steps
- Lack of play areas
- Dog fouling a greater issue than vandalism or violence
- Poor access to shops
- Poor bus service off estate
- Draughty, damp, cold housing

Socioeconomic environment
- Hard to manage financially
- 80% had central heating, but used by few owing to expense
- 90% of prescriptions were exempt
- 44% of the 16–19-year-olds were unemployed
- 37% of the 20–40-year-old males were unemployed

Disease and disability
- Perceived causes of ill-health: unemployment, stress, damp, poor diet and smoking
- Drug abuse among the young
- Social isolation among the elderly
- Needlestick injuries in children from rubbish
- Asthma, bronchitis, heart problems and arthritis
- Drug users were not concerned about HIV infection and not using condoms

- Domestic violence
- 20% of adults suffered from a long-term illness

Educational services
- Demand for after-school care, youth provision, adult education classes
- Good nearby youth project with activity groups and work for those who experience exceptional difficulties

Health services
- Long occupational therapy and chiropody waiting lists
- Shortage of district nurses and auxiliaries to help bathe
- It was sometimes hard to get an appointment with the local general practitioners
- Demand for telephone advice service
- There were worsening queues at the Accident and Emergency Department
- Poor discharge arrangements
- Ambulance transport problems
- Day centre for dementia appreciated by users

Social services
- Local social services were well known and appreciated
- Non-locally based services were not well known
- Lack of information led to under-utilization
- Shortage of home helps
- More support needed for carers

Health policy
- Little knowledge about the Patients' Charter and the Community Care Plan
- Health policy interventions thought to be cost-cutting exercises
- Concern about mentally ill 'being released into the community'

been implemented, were imminent or were under discussion at the completion of the initial appraisal. These are shown in Box 11.5.

Box 11.5 Immediate impact of rapid participatory appraisal

1. Lothian transport routed a bus through the estate
2. The city architect considered the creation of 'dog-free zones' in the estate
3. The Social Work Department arranged for the mental health development worker to run a community mental health group
4. Home help supervisor ran information in-service courses for home helps to inform clients of relevant services
5. The Community Education Department held introductory 'taster sessions' in complementary therapies
6. The local practice obtained toys for the waiting area and addressed older patients more formally, and encouraged local pharmacists to collect prescriptions for repeat medications
7. The local counsellors and a citizens' advice worker planned to hold regular surgeries
8. A local directory of community agencies established for PHCT
9. An information day planned

Most of the initiatives were established in the community room, fostering the sense of community, and many, such as the local practice activity, were in response to specific community feedback.

The study did not identify any previously unknown medical problems but the team obtained a deeper understanding of the health and social problems in the neighbourhood.

Conclusions

The *strengths* of rapid participatory appraisal are:

1. It is a multidisciplinary approach with workers from different sectors studying and learning together
2. It helps develop teamwork within the primary health care team
3. Development of the role of the user and community leaders and workers in evaluating and planning health care
4. It complements quantitative methods of assessing need
5. It emphasizes the place general practice has within the wider community and encourages community-oriented primary care
6. As an action research method it facilitates change; in the Dumbiedykes study, a neighbourhood profile was generated which collated needs, services, and suggestions for change.

The *drawbacks* of this method are:

1. It is a relatively new method, and thus training is necessary
2. Little quantitative information is obtained
3. The work is intense and it takes considerable time and

effort to listen and try to understand local people while at the same time explaining to them the professionals' way of looking at a problem
4. Coordination of a team may be logistically difficult
5. Funding may be necessary to secure recruitment of a relevant team.

In contrast to quantitative methods used by epidemiologists, rapid appraisal offers very specific insights, helping define what the problems are, rather than how many people are affected by problems. It helps identify the strength of feeling within the community on key issues.

Rapid appraisal provides a structure to elicit and learn from local opinions relatively easily. One attraction of such appraisal methods is their flexibility. Trained external researchers can be utilized, but in Dumbiedykes local workers undertaking the research had many advantages. Their knowledge of potentially available services was useful and ensured that when residents expressed a need which could be quickly resourced, exploration of that area was encouraged. A local directory of agencies in the community which contribute to the health of residents of Dumbiedykes was quickly established and increasingly used by the practice team. Local ownership of the research process means that the actions are more likely to be implemented.

We have used the opportunities to work jointly with the community to develop services to meet needs, and to facilitate team work between statutory and voluntary agencies. This community development approach in primary care may be more successful than community development projects that are more distant from the resources. A forum and mechanisms for giving patients access to the decision-making process are not just important in principle: they are also essential in practice if patients and the public are to be fully involved in their health care. Some Dumbiedykes residents now perceive their doctors as what Hart (1988) has called 'community general practitioners' and have commented positively on the doctors' public advocacy of 'healthy' policies.

Many of the findings had little medical content. Yet those responsible for other sectors have responded enthusiastically to suggestions from the community vocalized and supported by the extended primary care team. Rapid appraisal encourages a broad perspective on the health needs of individuals, and also helps doctors identify and enjoy a wider professional responsibility to the community. The jury is still out on what is professionally realistic for the new general practitioner in the networking nineties and beyond (Stott 1994). A further tested and modified rapid appraisal technique may be one important method of assessing health and social need in primary care.

COMMUNITY PROFILING

Introduction

Much work has been done in individual disciplines using single methods to assess need. In Chapter 4 the use of routine practice data is illustrated, and in Chapter 8 the use of patient surveys is described. Epidemiologically based needs assessment is described in Chapter 6, and the importance of factors outside the health sector is considered in Chapter 10. Little has been done to bring together these conceptually different approaches to create an overall multifaceted picture of need. Community profiling, however, is a set of techniques or an approach which has been utilized by many disciplines outside medicine, and by primary care workers in the developing countries to gather data from various sources to describe a community. Community profiling can use information from all the above sources to assess the needs, wants, demands and resources in a community. A community profile is a social, environmental and economic description of a given area which is used to inform local decision making (Burton 1994). The Health Visitors Association (Twinn et al 1992) and the Royal College of Nursing (1993) have both produced leaflets on profiling practice populations. However, profiling communities requires time and resources.

Process

To examine which approaches to community profiling might be most informative from a primary care base, a detailed community profile using a combination of the following methods and data sources was drawn up in a small neighbourhood, coordinated by a local general practitioner (Murray & Graham 1995).

Process 1 – rapid participatory appraisal. A multisectoral team comprising a local general practitioner, health visitor, two social workers, and community education worker collected information from existing documents about the neighbourhood, from interviews with a range of informants, and from direct observations of the neighbourhood. This has been described in greater detail in the previous section.

Process 2 – postal survey. A computer search was made listing patients of the researchers' practice who were aged over 16 years and who lived in Dumbiedykes. An output file was made and used with a mail merge facility to address and send the questionnaires. A questionnaire and a reply paid envelope was posted with a letter signed by the senior partner explaining confidentiality and giving brief details of the proposed survey. Four weeks later a reminder with a fresh questionnaire was sent to non-respondents. A mixture of lay concepts and medical diagnoses was used. It covered the following areas:

1. Chronic illness
2. Acute illnesses and experience of common symptoms
3. Health status – a standard multidimensional measure was included
4. Use of health services over 6 months
5. Perceived need for current and potential services
6. Social and demographic characteristics
7. Questions for people with long-term health problems, smokers and carers.

Process 3 – routinely available local statistics. Lothian Health Information and Statistics Unit provided information on hospital-based morbidity relating to the 19 postcodes for Dumbiedykes (population 1185) and for Lothian as a whole (population 726 010) for comparison. Complete data for 1991 were available. Data on births and deaths from the Registrar General for 1991 were also analysed. The 1991 census data were interrogated for the 19 postcodes that comprised Dumbiedykes.

Process 4 – practice-held information. Information was obtained on the Dumbiedykes residents registered with the study practice using the following methods:

1. Utilizing computerized records, the prevalence of chronic illness, repeat prescribing details and various screening and health promotion data were obtained
2. A random sample of 100 medical records was analysed, and the incidence of acute illness, acute prescribing and psychosocial problems was recorded
3. Referrals to hospitals and other agencies were examined for the previous year
4. A review of deaths in Dumbiedykes from 1991–94 was made
5. Surgery consultations, house calls, and out of hours visits were analysed
6. The registers of drug addicts and HIV patients were examined
7. Data were requested from the practice-attached community nurses.

Findings

The findings of the four processes are summarized in Box 11.6.

Box 11.7 highlights four conditions out of over 20 tabulated in the study: asthma/chronic bronchitis (a common physical illness), stress (the most common mental health problem), HIV/drug abuse (a particular problem in the neighbourhood) and smoking. Asthma/chronic bronchitis had a very high prevalence from the postal survey, a high prevalence from practice data, and few outpatient referrals were made, but this contribution was associated with a substantial number of admissions and several deaths. Eighteen per cent of respondents of the survey (rising to 26% of women aged 16–44 years) reported they

---

Box 11.6 Summary of findings of the processes used

Rapid participatory appraisal
- Little sense of community identity
- Hills, difficult steps, lack of play areas for children
- Financial hardship
- Perceived causes of ill health included unemployment, stress, dampness, poor diet and eating habits, and smoking
- Drug misuse amongst some young people
- Social isolation among the elderly people
- Asthma, bronchitis, heart problems, and arthritis were common
- Long waiting lists for occupational therapy and chiropody
- Shortage of district nurses and auxiliaries to help with personal hygiene
- Sometimes hard to get an appointment with local general practitioners
- The most important health needs were for a bus into the estate; play areas for toddlers; activities in the community room and a local supermarket.

Postal survey (62% response rate)
- Mainly gastrointestinal and musculoskeletal problems
- Over 65-year-olds scored worse on the Nottingham Health Profile pain and physical mobility subscales
- 16–44 year age group scored worse on the emotional reaction and social isolation subscales
- Advice about medication, stress, heart disease, smoking, welfare benefits and healthy eating needed

Routine statistics (%)

	Dumbiedykes	Lothian
Census		
Over age 50 years	42	30
Male unemployment	26	11
Owner occupier	20	60
Car owner	15	54
Limiting long-term illness	20	12
Hospital		
Outpatient attendance	14	13
Births to single mothers	41	25
Midtrimester abortions or % of local births	14	<1
Common procedures	IV chemotherapy Endoscopy HIV treatment	Endoscopy Cystoscopy Abortion

Practice held data
- Musculoskeletal, nervous and gastrointestinal systems commonest problems
- Acute illness caused much workload
- Dumbiedykes's patients had an excess of psychosocial problems
- Patient contact with the primary health care team was 7.3 per patient per year
- Highest prescribing costs related to the gastrointestinal system with 3.3% of patients on acid suppressants
- The community nurses held considerable data about infants, the housebound and the elderly which was not being routinely shared in the team

---

had trouble with stress, depression or 'bad nerves'. However, stress was only documented in 12% of medical records. Census data revealed high unemployment, many single parents and other potential stressers, and the appraisal gave unique insights into the lives of individuals. Substantial data about drug users and HIV in

Dumbiedykes and smoking were revealed by each method. In general, unique information was provided by each method. Except for the traditional use of hospital information, all methods of appraisal showed that the most prevalent conditions in the community were arthritis, gastrointestinal problems and stress or depression, a finding which rings true in daily general practice.

Advantages and disadvantages of individual methods

Rapid participatory appraisal encouraged a broad multi-disciplinary approach to assessing health need. The role of selected users, community leaders and workers in prioritizing and planning care was developed. A neighbourhood profile was generated which detailed needs, available resources and contained suggestions for change. The process in itself facilitated change. Because people's broad priorities were heard, health service interventions were weighed against other options to improve the quality of life locally.

The postal survey yielded detailed information about acute and chronic illness, and perceived need for existing and potential services for both users and non-users. The instrument could be reapplied to the same population or to a different population for comparisons over time or across areas. Individual community members identified their own needs. However, respondents were less likely to raise their own agendas and there was a low response rate in young men. Considerable time, resources and specific skills were again required.

Routine local statistics gave a descriptive account of morbidity and socioeconomic indicators and allowed comparison with regional norms. Collaboration between public health and primary care allowed sharing of perspectives and skills, and permitted comparison of ward-based and practice-based data sets.

Practice data collection facilitated teamwork. Much information was available from computerized data, medical records, annual reports and financial statements, but this had to be analysed and 'cleaned'. Much local knowledge of the neighbourhood was implicit, and was explicitly documented with some effort.

Impact

In Dumbiedykes, the participative appraisal was the only method which brought about change during the data collection process itself. This was due to the community involvement. The major findings of each method were presented to the practice management team at Mackenzie Medical Centre when they were drawing up their 1995 business plan. The following issues were considered important:

- Arthritis, gastrointestinal problems and stress were the most common problems of the patients

Box 11.7   Collation of findings of the different methods

	Practical data	Local statistics	Postal survey	Rapid appraisal
Asthma/ Chronic Bronchitis	6.5% prevalence 6% on bronchodilators 3% on inhaled steroids	Few outpatient referrals 13% of all admissions 3 deaths	14% prevalence 9% seen doctor in last 6 months for this	'Many toiling for breath' Damp housing causes asthma in children
Stress/ Depression	12% (medical records search) Medical records of 100 non-respondents to the postal survey reported stress/depression in 20, drug misuse in 8 and alcohol problems in 6.	Census revealed many potential stressers: high unemployment many single parents.	18% prevalence of being anxious/depressed/bad nerves. 10% seen doctor in last 6 months for this. 72% requested help or advice. 16–44 age group scored highly on NHP on emotional reaction and social isolation sub-scales. A help-line with someone who will listen to you was suggested.	Stressful environment and lifestyles. Regular Citizen's Advice, a course about alternative therapies, and a crèche were suggested.
Drugs Users/ HIV	Many patients on methadone substitution therapy lived in Dumbiedykes. High turnover of drug addicts. Several children with needlestick injuries. Moving out of Dumbiedykes was the solution some patients gave for their drug problem.	HIV carrier was the fifth most common reason for adult hospital admission in 1991. Many indicators of socioeconomic disadvantage revealed by census.	6% wanted help or advice about illegal drugs. 26% wanted help or advice about HIV. 'Would like HIV test without documentation' – freetext.	Interviews revealed a broad and detailed picture. Some young families and socially isolated single parents were abusing drugs. Drug users received prescribed substitutes and also bought extra medication from suppliers within Dumbiedykes. Drug users were not concerned about HIV infection and even the few who still injected were not using condoms. Domestic violence was common. Most residents old and young alike knew of drug users and many commented: 'This used to be a really nice area.' Needles found by residents in bin stores.
Smoking	50% current smokers. Many smokers had died of smoking related diseases.	Frequent admissions for disorders of the circulatory and respiratory systems. High smoking related mortality.	47% current smokers. 50% of smokers want help or advice about giving up. Opportunistic advice is the most popular method of health promotion.	Smoking a perceived cause of ill health in the community but a necessary coping mechanism or just a habit. More young girls smoke. 30% of the local shop's turnover was for cigarettes.

- A high 'therapeutic' abortion rate existed locally and in Edinburgh
- Twice as many people considered they had heart problems and asthma than had been formally diagnosed
- Affluent and deprived communities were served by the practice.

A number of interventions were suggested. However, the incentive-linked disease management programme for diabetes and asthma, and the remunerative health promotion work, were considered current priorities, due to the national guidelines and payments. No extra time or resources could be made available for the above and other areas of high locally identified expressed need, apart from a zero-cost family planning initiative. An initiative to address the most common problems presenting to the general practitioners was clearly desirable, and would potentially benefit three large relatively neglected groups of patients as well as possibly decreasing the consultation rate. The considerable impact of carrying out the rapid participatory appraisal has already been described.

Conclusions

– the ability of methods to tackle different issues

Different methods yielded complementary insights into health needs generally, and into specific problems. With asthma/chronic bronchitis and ischaemic heart disease (examples of ongoing physical problems), practice data and survey data had the greatest utility. The problems of drug abuse and HIV in the community were best revealed by rapid appraisal and data collection within the practice, a combination also found useful to explore other psychosocial issues. The postal survey usefully supplemented practice data about acute illness within the community. Inpatient admissions compared with the rest of Lothian provided a proxy of need for secondary care. The postal survey was able to display a different frequency of perceived and formally diagnosed illness. The context of health service provision was best informed by the appraisal and census data. Indeed, a more immediate need for 'non-health' services than 'health' services was vocalized by the appraisal.

Community involvement in health is an important issue, both as a democratic goal in itself and as a potentially useful means of achieving an improvement in health. The extent of public involvement in these methods, in decreasing order, was: rapid appraisal (where providers and patients interacted and learnt from each other); postal survey (when respondents' perceptions and suggestions were read and analysed); practice data gathered by a team in daily contact with patients over many years; and routine statistics supplied without any patient involvement. Rapid appraisal ensured that the voices of patients and community leaders were heard directly. To give people an effective voice in the shaping of health services locally will call for a radically different approach from that employed in the past (NHS Management Executive 1992).

SUMMARY

Within general practice, lack of planning time and the pressure to respond to the immediate needs of patients lead to local studies about health status and health care needs being given low priority. A coherent, practical, explicit and multifaceted approach is required to assess need for community-based, primary and hospital health care services. This chapter has presented three overlapping approaches to needs assessment. Caution must be exercised when using only a single method or technique, as many researchers have done in the past. Practice data may understate the prevalence of disease in the community. Postal surveys should be interpreted carefully, especially when doctors and patients may understand words such as hypertension differently. A small number of in-depth interviews does not set out to sample a representative section of the study population. A few unusual events may skew very small area statistics. Inpatient admissions for most diagnoses are not a proxy for morbidity in the community (Payne et al 1994). Results are likely to be more relevant if data from one source are checked against data from at least two other sources. All major definitions of good general practice refer to the need to consider physical, psychological and social well-being.

The work described in this chapter employed different approaches in gathering data to understand the composition and needs of a community. A holistic assessment of health and health service needs obtained by such techniques is most likely to identify effective interventions.

APPENDIX 1. INTERVIEWING SCHEDULE

1. *Community composition*
   How long have you lived here?
   Do you know your neighbours?
   Do you have friends or relatives in this area that you see often?
   Can you describe the kinds of people who live in this area?
   Is the area better for some people to live in rather than others?

2. *Socioeconomic environment*
   Are you aware of many people who find it hard to manage financially?
   How would you describe your own financial situation?
   Does your financial situation cause you any particular difficulties?
   How often do you go out ... shopping ... socializing?
   I'm sure you've heard reports on the TV and in the newspapers about domestic violence? Do you know if domestic violence is a problem in this area?

3. *Community organization and structure*
   Do you know of any special organizations for the residents of Dumbiedykes?
   Can you think of any community activities which would be helpful to people in this area?

4. *Community capacity*
   Do you know of any local people who are good at getting things done?
   Do you think there is a sense of community identity and/or commitment to this area?
   Do you feel part of the community?

5. *Physical environment*
   Are there any particular problems with living in this area?
   How would you describe the condition of the housing in Dumbiedykes?
   Are there any particular problems with your house/flat?
   Does transport or access to the area present you with any problems?
   How safe do you feel in the neighbourhood, e.g. walking outside after dark or being at home alone? If not why?
   Are you aware of any environmental health problems in the area?

6. *Disease and disability profile*
   What do you think are the worst health problems in the area?
   Have these changed over the last few years?
   Do you know if drug abuse is a problem?
   Do you know if alcohol abuse is a problem?
   Are there many people with a physical or learning disability living in the area?

7. *Educational services*
   Are you aware of these services available locally? [*prompt list*]
   How could they be improved?
   Is there anything else you would like in the area?

8. *Health services*
   Which of these medical services do you or have you used? [*prompt list*]
   What is the best thing about them and what could be better?
   Do you have any suggestions that would help to improve these services?
   What do you think of hospital services?
   Which hospital services do you use?
   Have you noticed any recent changes in these services?

9. *Social services*
   What social services do you use?
   What social services do people in the area use?
   What do you think of them?
   How would you like to see them improved?

10. *Healthy policy*
    There have been recent changes in the Health and Social Work Policy. Have you received any of the following leaflets: [*show leaflets*]

    Patients Charter   Community Care Plan

    Have you read them?
    Patients Charter   Community Care Plan
    Do you think they will change anything?

11. *Miscellaneous*
    If you could wave a magic wand, what changes would you like to make in the area?
    Thinking about yourself and your family, has there ever been a time when you thought that help was not there when you needed it?
    Would you know where to get help?
    Is there anything you would like to ask or add?

APPENDIX 2. LIST OF KEY INFORMANTS

1. Voluntary Worker, St Ann's Community Centre
2. Visiting Sister, St Patrick's RC Church
3. Home Care Organizer, Social Work Department
4. Project Director, South Side Care Project
5. Dumbiedykes Social Club Convenor
6. Local Lothian Regional Councillors
7. Project Co-ordinator, Safer Edinburgh Project
8. Local District Counsellors
9. Local Community Involvement Policeman
10. Receptionist, Mackenzie Medical Centre
11. Community Development Worker
12. Old Town Renewal Trust
13. Housing Department Officer, Edinburgh District Council
14. Pharmacist
15. Local District Nurse
16. Head Teacher and Deputy Head Teacher, Local Primary School
17. Volunteer, Women's Royal Voluntary Service
18. Community Psychiatric Nurse, Community Drug Problems Service
19. Shopkeeper, Dumbiedykes Store
20. Project Co-ordinator, Local Youth Project
21. Local Health Visitor
22. Public Transport Unit, Planning Department, Lothian Regional Council
23. Co-ordinator, Dumbiedykes Children's Centre
24. Recently retired local general practitioner
25. Group interview – Board of Directors of South Side Care Project
26. Group interview – Reminiscence Group
27. Group interview – Dumbiedykes Residents Association
28. Group discussion – teenage girls at a youth project

REFERENCES

Brody H 1992 Philosophic approaches. In: Crabtree B, Miller W (eds) Doing qualitative research: multiple strategies. Sage Publications, London

Burton P 1994 Community profiling. A guide to identifying needs. University of Bristol School of Advanced Urban Studies, Bristol

Cresswell T 1992 Assessing community health and social needs in north Derbyshire using participatory rapid appraisal. Medical Sociology News 17(3): 27–38

Department of Health 1994 Department of Health Register of Cost-effectiveness Studies. Economics and Operational Research Division, Department of Health, London

Gillam S, Plamping D, McClenahan J et al 1994 Community-oriented primary care. King's Fund, London

Hart J T 1988 A new kind of doctor. Merlin Press, London

Institute of Medicine 1984 Community-oriented primary care: a practical assessment. National Academic Press, Washington, DC, vol 1

Johnson J C 1990 Selecting ethnographic informants. Sage, London

Kark S L 1974 From medicine in the community to community medicine. Journal of the American Medical Association 228: 1585–1586

Kark S L 1981 Community-oriented primary health care. Appleton Century-Crofts, New York

Manderson L, Aaby P 1992 An epidemic in the field? Rapid assessment procedures & health research. Social Science and Medicine 35(7): 839–850

Murray S A 1995. A critical assessment of the use of rapid participatory appraisal to assess health needs in a small neighbourhood. MD Thesis, Aberdeen University

Murray S A, Graham L J C 1995 Practice based health needs assessment: use of four methods in a small neighbourhood. British Medical Journal 310: 1443–1448

Murray S A, Tapson J, Turnbull L, McCallum J, Little A 1994 Listening to local voices: adapting rapid appraisal to assess health and social needs in a general practice. British Medical Journal 308: 698–700

NHS Management Executive 1992 Local voices. The views of local people in purchasing for health. Department of Health, London

Ong B N, Humphris G, Annett H, Rifkin S 1991 Rapid appraisal in an urban setting, an example from the developed world. Social Science and Medicine 32(8): 909–915

Payne J N, Coy J, Patterson S, Milner P C 1994 Is use of hospital services a proxy for morbidity? A small area comparison of the prevalence of arthritis, depression, dyspepsia, obesity, and respiratory disease with inpatient admission rates for these disorders in England. Journal of Epidemiology and Community Health 48: 74–78

Pickles W 1939 Epidemiology in county practice. John Wright, Bristol (Republished 1994 Royal College of General Practitioners, London)

Royal College of Nursing 1993 The GP practice population profile: a framework for every member of the primary health care team. Royal College of Nursing, London

Stott N C H 1994 The new general practitioner? British Medical Journal 44: 2–3

Toon P 1994 What is good general practice? Occasional paper 65. Royal College of General Practitioners, London

Twinn S, Dauncey J, Carnell J 1992 The process of health profiling. Health Visitors' Association, London

Welbourne A 1992 Rapid rural notes 16. Special issue on applications for health. International Institute for Environment and Development, London

World Health Organization 1995 Guidelines for rapid participatory appraisal to assess community health needs. WHO, Geneva

Information and conclusions

12

The collection and interpretation of information

Yvonne Doyle

INTRODUCTION

Information is the servant of decision making. If collected and used appropriately, information can guide good professional practice. However, the quest to gather information for its own sake or for an anonymous third party with no feedback to the searcher quickly becomes a time-wasting tyranny. In the busy general practice setting, it is important that any work involving the collection of information is undertaken with a clear purpose in view. 'Needs analysis' is not necessarily such a purpose. The term is vague and is used to signify an often lengthy process, which may not have a defined outcome at the start, i.e. a precise answer to the question: 'A need for what?'

There are three questions which are worth asking at the outset of undertaking a needs analysis exercise in the practice setting. These are:

● What am I trying to achieve by conducting this needs analysis?
● Who will be the main user(s) of the information collected?
● Who will be the beneficiaries of the exercise?

This calls for pause to consider the links between the process and the outcome of needs analysis, linking the public health, information, clinical practice, and managerial aspects of the exercise. All of these aspects are relevant to the practice in undertaking a needs analysis, and in this order of progress. The public health considerations within the practice setting will define the questions being addressed in undertaking the analysis; an intelligent information collection will follow; and the results will guide clinical practice and managerial action within the practice.

CHECKLISTS IN ADVANCE OF COLLECTING INFORMATION FOR A NEEDS ANALYSIS

There are at least four users of information collected at practice level. These potential users are the practice itself (or individual champions within the practice); managers of a locality or general practice multifund where the practice is located; the district health authority or local health service management; and national research and data collection projects (Drever 1994, Griffin et al 1994, de Grauw et al 1995). In the first three of these cases, the information collected is frequently for a needs analysis exercise, with the aim of informing purchasing of care by or for the practice; the allocation of resources to practices; the comparison of variations in care; or as a guide to the provision of services by practices in future. Beyond the practice level, health authorities and regional and national programmes may aim to use the information to examine epidemiological and service utilization variations, and the links with the economics of priority setting and resource allocation.

Whoever uses the information eventually it is assumed here that the collection of information will be undertaken by members of the general practice. For those embarking on a needs analysis at practice level, addressing the questions in the checklist in Box 12.1 may be useful.

Table 12.1 will prompt consideration of the type of needs analysis to be undertaken. The most desirable type for an individual practice undertaking the exercise for its own purposes is that which will allow for the required action without a large investment in new data collection. This is particularly relevant in the context of the validity and reliability of information collected from primary care sources, and will be dealt with later on in

---

Box 12.1 Ten questions about resources to consider in advance of a needs analysis in general practice

1. Why is this work being undertaken?
2. Who will lead the exercise?
3. Who will do the work?
4. Has a similar exercise been undertaken elsewhere, and can this be accessed and used?
5. If not, are the skills present in this practice to lead and undertake the work?
6. Should outside help be sought, and what type of help would complement in-house skills?
7. What other resources are needed in the practice to do the work?
8. How can the cost to the practice be minimized?
9. What detail and accuracy of information is needed?
10. Are data protection and confidentiality likely to be relevant in this exercise?

---

this chapter. In addition to this, it is worth considering some general technical questions about the needs analysis before embarking on the collection of information. This will save time during the work, guiding collection of appropriate information and analysis. Table 12.1 summarizes these questions.

TYPES OF INFORMATION FOR NEEDS ANALYSIS

It is helpful to view the variety of information available towards needs analysis in three broad categories: statistical and epidemiological; sources of evidence-based information (mainly textual); and qualitative, such as from surveys and research. The largest group is the first, and much needs analysis is based solely on statistical and epidemiological profiles of the population of interest. Table 12.2 shows the source of these groups of information, how readily available and the local or wider

---

Table 12.1 Technical questions and answers about the purpose and progress of the needs analysis

Question	Possible options
What is the precise question being addressed in this exercise/what need is being analysed?	An epidemiological profile of the practice
	A purchasing profile of the practice
	A determination of unmet need through the proxy of service utilization
	A determination of equity of service distribution within the practice population
	A comparison of effectiveness within the practice with accepted 'good' practice
	A canvass of patients about their perception of need
What type of information might inform this?	Statistical data
	Secondary statistical sources (e.g. annual public health reports)
	Clinical and managerial 'intelligence' (local, national and international)
	Results of statistical and qualitative published surveys
	Collection of new information (quantitative or qualitative)
What aspects of the information chosen need consideration?	Where can the information be accessed?
	Is it held manually or computerized? Is it in the public domain, and at no charge?
	Is the information current, complete and accurate?
	Are the definitions and presentation of data standardized? Is the information comparable across populations, time periods and geographical boundaries?
Will the results of this exercise aid decision making?	Action can be taken with the strategic use of readily available information (either tailor made or from aggregated sources)
	A new data collection exercise is needed

relevance of the source. This table is not exhaustive but is an example of the range of information available.

For a busy practice, the easiest route to the statistical information may be to use secondary sources, particularly the annual public health report of the local director of public health. The district health authority is likely to have access to analysis on local and national epidemiological, demographic and service utilization data which would be useful to the practice as a comparator or to provide denominator data. The information alluded to in Table 12.2 is of variable quality. For example research on the use of prescribing data in the UK as a proxy for other variables has concluded that, although promising, prescribing data use needs further research (Davis et al 1994). It has also been found that diagnoses and the practitioner's style exert considerable influence on prescribing variations in primary care (Lloyd et al 1995). An investigation of general practice annual reports has identified that more standardized data need to be collected before interpractice comparisons could be undertaken using this source (Record et al 1994). The interpretation of service utilization data is complex, and variations in utilization occur for a myriad of reasons other than morbidity in the underlying populations (Wennberg & Gittlesohn 1973). Two sources of information deserve mention due to their wide use and versatility.

Census data

The census provides a wide range of primary statistical data and much further analysis and compilation of useful local profiles and indicators (such as deprivation indices, and epidemiological profiles, down to the small area level). Analysis of trends between two sets of census by researchers from the Office of Population Censuses and Surveys (OPCS) in the UK has provided important socioeconomic and epidemiological information at the national level about groups of interest in the population (for example children, families and minority ethnic groups) (Office of Population Censuses and Surveys, 1995). The census has also been used to monitor and promote equity in the uptake of primary care. Data from existing child health information services have been combined with census data for small areas to show wide variations in uptake of preventive services between affluent and deprived communities (Majeed et al 1994a). The census has also been used to explain variations in uptake of primary care (Majeed et al 1994b), and to predict actual resource requirements in general practice (Majeed 1995). A familiarity with the range of census data available and the local work under way using the census is likely to be time well spent for those pursuing analysis at a practice level.

National evidence-based networks

The Cochrane Centre and the Centre for Reviews and Dissemination have been set up to investigate and promote the use of effective clinical interventions. The work of the two programmes complements each other (Sheldon & Chalmers 1994). The output is heavily used by health authority purchasers and policy makers in the UK. The information provided is deliberately user-friendly and will provide the most authoritative information available in the specific areas in which work has been conducted.

AT WHAT LEVEL CAN PRACTICES ENGAGE IN NEEDS ASSESSMENT?

Examples in the UK show that there are two ways in which a practice engages with needs assessment exercises. The practice may gather and use the information purely for the purposes of that practice; and the practice may be part of a wider project, usually run in conjunction with the district health authority to which the practice may contribute its own information.

Practices which use information for their own purposes may use information from their own practice, or a range of information as in Table 12.2 from other sources. The practice sources which are frequently used are:

- Age–sex data from the practice register
- Indicators of risk from preventive medical services
- Date of registration and mobility of patients
- Disease-specific information, for example from disease registers
- Service utilization within primary care and to secondary care (such as referrals)
- Prescribing patterns
- Mortality within the practice population
- Occasionally, special practice surveys, usually conducted by a member of the team other than the general practitioner
- Occasionally, focus groups, questionnaires and other systematic feedback from users of the practice.

If practices in an area are considering embarking on contributing to a wider programme of local data collection towards needs analysis, it may be helpful to know of some examples of similar schemes in the UK. All of these schemes involve sharing information between primary care and other agencies, usually including the district health authority, in a computerized relationship which allows feedback to practices with their own and comparative data.

One of these schemes is the Medics programme (Murphy & Jenkins 1995). Medics is a collaborative project between Northumberland Health Authority and 33 practices with a combined population of 222 000 in

Table 12.2 Examples of information types and sources for needs assessment

Type of information	Description of source	Local and wider location of source(s)
Demography, statistical	Population registers Births, stillbirths, infant deaths Census data GP age–sex registers and list size Deprivation indices	District health authority Local postgraduate library Local health authority, via census databases and the Public Health Common Data Set in the UK Regional perinatal monitoring groups in the UK Practice data District health authority
Annual reports, statistical and textual, range of data types	Chief Medical Officer, national Director of public health, district level Practice annual reports	Local postgraduate library District health authority Local practices
Mortality, statistical	Local deaths at electoral ward level, available as OPCS publication in UK Practice registers and recorded activity	Local postgraduate library District health authority including the Public Health Common Data Set Extracts in annual public health reports Local practices
Morbidity, statistical	Screening and vaccination/immunization statistics Cancer registrations Communicable disease epidemiology General household survey (self-determined illness) National morbidity surveys in sample general practices Special registers (e.g. congenital malformations, OPCS) Disease registers at practice level Child health surveillance Prescribing data, PACT returns	District health authority, local practices Cancer registries Public Health Laboratory System (UK) Local postgraduate library, health authority E.g. RCGP Unit, Birmingham; Continuous Morbidity Registration, Nijmegen National and regional sources; district health authority Local practices District health authority, local health visitors District health authority
Morbidity, statistical ('comparative needs assessment')	Activity data from health service utilization *Primary care*: – Risk factor profiles from preventive service use – Activity data in primary care – Referral data to secondary care *Secondary care* (local and national): – Attendances at ambulatory care – Admission rates by speciality – Discharge diagnoses – Contact rates with community services – Use of genitourinary services – Use of family planning services	District health authority and local practices District health authority; individual hospitals and community services; information units of academic units and public health institutes
Broader determinants of health, statistical and qualitative ('corporate needs assessment')	Social services profiles of services to population groups Information relating to housing type and repair Environmental health information Local probation service and police statistics Local accident data Community activities of the religious organizations Profiles undertaken by voluntary groups	Relevant local authority departments Relevant local religious organizations Relevant local voluntary agencies
Evidence-based information	Information on effective care for selected various conditions (e.g. stroke, breast cancer, epilepsy) Information on recommended effective interventions in selected circumstances (e.g. use of guidelines, cholesterol testing, health promotion) Outcomes briefings Health Technology Assessment via the NHS R&D Programme (UK) UK NHS Regional purchaser briefings (e.g. *Bandolier*) Getting Research Into Practice (the GRIP Project)	Cochrane Centres via the international Cochrane Collaborations Centre for Reviews and Dissemination at the University of York, UK Centre for Reviews and Dissemination at the University of York, UK Institute of Public Health, Wessex *Bandolier* information from Oxford Regional Health Authority Oxford Regional Health Authority
Local/regional surveys and qualitative information	Health status questionnaire surveys Consumer satisfaction (e.g. by local consumer groups) Local research surveys (e.g. on patient follow-up status) Public health pages on the Internet	Health authority, postgraduate library, source of the survey Appropriate pages of the Internet special interest groups (quality variable!)

Northumberland. The aims of the project are to assist the health authority in the task of purchasing; and to assist general practices in understanding the health characteristics of their registered population. The emphasis of the project is to improve the quality of general practice information. Data are collected from the practices in three general categories: chronic disease, risk factors, and data from screening of people aged over 75 years. Table 12.3 shows the variables collected in each of these categories.

The data are used for a wide range of purposes including epidemiological profiling of the population; monitoring of the National Health Strategy targets, practice parameters such as referral rates and consultation rates, and purchasing intelligence. The NHS Executive Information Management Group and the Northern Regional Health Authority have provided funding for the development of a software which could extract and format information from any general practice computer system using a Health Query Language. This development is called the *MIQUEST* scheme. *MIQUEST* is now used to extract data from half of the participating practices, and has reduced the input time for practice staff, while improving the reliability and repeatability of the data provided (Allan 1994). The data are presented in three forms: observed cases, crude rates and standardized morbidity ratios. The last statistical analysis allows comparison between practices with different population structures. Practices receive feedback with crude rates and standardized ratios, and may compare their statistics with other practices (which are anonymous).

DISP III (Liverpool University 1995) is a collaborative project between three health authorities, the Departments of General Practice and Public Health, Liverpool University, and primary health care teams in Liverpool. The purpose of the project is to collect accurate morbidity data from primary health care which are used to inform commissioning of health care. There are three types of information collected: core data, disease-specific data, and patient pathways in the health service.

*Morbidity Information Query and Export SynTax.

Core data include age–sex breakdown, indicators of risk, date of registration with the practice, and postcodes. Information on ethnic group was sought, but it proved difficult to yield much on this from routinely recorded practice data. Deprivation levels were thought to be a desirable variable, and although various components were discussed, it was also difficult to obtain these data from every practice. Morbidity data from practices, treatment, referral patterns, secondary care, and outcomes have been collected. The latter have been catered for by allowing free text in the computerized record to encourage recording a wide variety of outcomes. Disease-specific information has been collected on mental health, coronary heart disease, cancer, diabetes, back pain, accident and emergency referrals for minor injuries, and peptic ulcers. There were six levels recorded in relation to patient care, from management in primary care to treatment in other sectors, and one level is a field for qualitative information on outcomes. Particular attention has been paid to the organization and management data gathering, including the issues of data validity, reliability and repeatability. The method used was to create a new post, the data practice manager, in the primary health care team. The aims of the post included the collection and validation of relevant data, paying due attention to confidentiality, to engage in training and audit, and to undertake occasional local surveys.

The *LAPIS* 2 project in Sheffield is a collaborative project between Sheffield Health Authority and general practices, designed to gather data from disparate sources such as the family health service authority register, hospital inpatient events, the census, mortality data and health visiting profiles of the population (Sheffield Health Authority 1994). The purpose of the project is to support a more sophisticated understanding of the needs and challenges that practices and localities face in purchasing and providing care. LAPIS 2 uses two different sets of indicators: practice and ward indicators. There are 50 practice indicators, including those relating to the practice population and the utilization of primary and secondary care services by attenders at the practices. The ward indicators use census, mortality and service utilization variables. Information is presented as rates,

Table 12.3   The variables for which age–sex prevalence data are collected at 6 monthly intervals as part of the Medics scheme

Chronic disease	Health	Disability (over 75 years of age only)
Asthma	Alcohol consumption	Vision
Cancer[a]	Tobacco consumption	Hearing
Cerebrovascular disease	Blood pressure	Mobility
Diabetes	Body mass index	Continence
Hypertension		Cerebral functioning
Ischaemic heart disease		

[a]This variable will include cancers relevant to the local health strategy.

and in ranking order, and is menu driven so that a variety of data presentations can be chosen.

The Somerset Morbidity Project (Somerset Health 1995) is a continuous recording of morbidity in general practice. The project was set up in 1994, and by the end of 1995 there were 12 participating practices (out of 74) with a patient population of 78 000. The practices have been selected to be representative of the county of Somerset. The project aims to collect a valid and complete set of continuously updated morbidity information in order to inform and puruse evidence-based commissioning of both primary and secondary care. The project has concentrated on the collection of data which are useful to the secondary care sector, which helps to examine the quality of care in general practice, and explores whether it is possible to use the data to contract for unmet need in registered populations.

The project is a collaboration between Somerset Health Authority and general practices. The practices collect primary epidemiological information such as incidence, prevalence and disease trends on all contacts with the general practitioner using Read-coded diagnoses and consultation rates with type of consultation. Data are transmitted from practices weekly. Validation of the data are undertaken quarterly. Overall, 97% of the consultations on the validation days have been recorded on computer. Practices are paid a small honorarium for the time spent in producing weekly reports.

The project produces epidemiological data for practices with comparative trends, and various reports. Examples of 14 conditions reported in detail in previous reviews include:

- Allergic rhinitis
- Asthma
- Depression
- Glue ear
- Stroke
- Angina
- Back disorders
- Major mental illness
- Heart failure
- Diabetes
- Infertility
- Hypertension
- Tonsillitis/pharyngitis
- Urinary incontinence.

These and other conditions chosen represented high cost and volume to the health authority, topical clinical issues, and the need to respond to provider proposals. Two recent examples of topics which were dealt with in detail are evidence-based purchasing for patients with angina, and the problem of unmet need in relation to urinary incontinence (Somerset Health and Somerset Family Health Authority 1995). In the case of angina, a particular interest of the health authority was to predict the appropriate surgical intervention rate for operative interventions such as coronary artery bypass grafts. This was estimated by combining information about the local incidence of angina, and literature sources on the accuracy of diagnosis and the expected benefit from the intervention (Somerset Health and Somerset Family Health Authority 1995). The morbidity data have also been used to compare prescribing patterns across Somerset practices in relation to health need as expressed by morbidity. The conclusion that variations in prescribing could not be accounted for solely by variations in morbidity led to the further suggestion that the participating practices could use the results for their internal clinical audit. Morbidity reviews are produced by the project team on a half-yearly basis. A major problem with most morbidity surveys, including the National GP morbidity surveys and the GP Weekly Returns Service, is that in relying on volunteer practices they are subject to selection bias. The Somerset project has addressed this by only selecting a group of practices which are representative of the entire county. But by choosing recording of GPs' perception rather than conformation with strict criteria, the measures of morbidity may be more subject to variance in reliability than other surveys.

A collaborative project between Bromley Health Authority and local general practices has led to the *Bromley Health Phased Approach* to Needs Assessment in Primary Care (Pearson & Barker 1995). The project aims to develop a practice profile which can be standardized as an approach for all practices, based on available data manipulated to be practice relevant. The potential of these data to inform resource allocation based on health care need is being explored. The sources of data include census, screening, commissioning, provider utilization, social services, and local survey data, combined with information from general practices such as practice demography, risk factor data, repeat prescribing, population mobility, disease-specific information, and elderly care information.

These projects are developmental, and have raised a number of issues which are relevant to the collection and interpretation of information either by the practice in isolation or as part of a wider project.

SOME ISSUES TO CONSIDER IN THE COLLECTION, INTERPRETATION AND USE OF INFORMATION

Data quality

Quality of data covers several issues. The first issue is the completeness and accuracy of the data. Completeness involves a systematic and regular check on the sources of the data for the coverage of the relevant topic or population. For example, large proportions of service utilization data may be missing due to lack of recording or poor coding. Aspects of practice data such as advice given on smoking may not be recorded in patient notes (Wilson & McDonald 1994). At a minimum, the scale of the absent data must be appreciated. Data accuracy should be checked also, for example by sampling the consistency of data entry and coding. The Medics project has joined with the local Medical Audit Advisory Group to conduct a formal assay of data and diagnostic accuracy.

The reliability of measurements or data relates to whether the same result or reading is obtained every time the data are collected and entered or the measurement is undertaken. A reliable result will be obtained if there is minimal or no variation in the process of measurement, collection and entry. Sources of variation come for example from the *same* data collector assigning different classification codes to a particular disease on different occasions (within-observer variation); from *different* data collectors on the same or different occasions (between-observer variation); and, in the case of surveys, the subjects/patients may generate their own variations. Instrument variation in this context may come, for example, from a questionnaire with biased or imprecise questions; thus the importance where possible of using previously validated survey instruments.

A further aspect of data quality relates to the alertness of the data collector for the validity of the data. Validity means that the result reflects what the observer set out to measure, giving the observer a 'true picture' of the topic of interest. A practice manager may wish to examine whether the practice has achieved a good uptake of a particular service. An examination of the number of patients in a time period who received the service as a proportion of those eligible could be undertaken. This might not be a valid measure if the denominator, the eligible practice population, was inaccurate. This was addressed recently in east London where an 'active patient denominator' was produced by excluding patients who were likely to have died, moved away, or who for administrative reasons were unable to contribute to the numerator (Robson & Falshaw 1995).

Standardization of information

Several project leaders involved in the collection of data in general practice have remarked that it is difficult to interpret outputs from general practice in the absence of standard protocols for the definition, collection, collation and presentation of data from general practice. Read coding has not necessarily alleviated coding problems because of between-observer variation in the coding of similar conditions.

Interpretation of interpractice variations

This presents a particular challenge. Two practices in the same vicinity may appear to have very different prevalences of a condition such as asthma. Is this because of a true difference in the prevalence of the condition in the attending populations; greater diagnostic accuracy of one practice in defining the condition; a drift of affected patients towards one practice which may have a special interest in the condition; a systematic error in one (or both) practice(s) in the coding of respiratory conditions; or simple random variation? Those interpreting these variations who work in general practice have an advantage over the distant observer due to their local knowledge, so long as they do not accept unusual variations at face value.

Data protection and confidentiality

It is well to check with a local senior information officer or a data custodian in the UK (under the Data Protection Act) about the protocol for access to certain data and protection of the rights of the individuals on whom the data are based, particularly if research or publication of sensitive information is envisaged. In the UK, many local ethics committees will insist on seeing a protocol if data on individual patients, including community-based data, are to be used for research or related activities.

Skills required to undertake the work

In large-scale projects where data are being collected for a district or national programme, some areas have trained individuals within the practice as data managers (Liverpool University 1995). This person is usually a practice administrator or manager, and the skills found useful to impart include communication, data validation and management, and basic epidemiology. As data collection becomes a more consuming aspect of practice life, the designation and training of a person as a practice data manager may represent resources well invested.

To survey or not to survey?

To answer this question, the practice team need to ask another: 'What will a survey provide for us that cannot be gleaned from other sources?' Outside of research settings, the number of situations absolutely requiring a survey are very limited, and a surprising amount of insight can be had from existing sources of information. It is even possible that a similar survey done elsewhere on a broadly similar population would be sufficient to use as an indicator. If the practice decides to survey, the best option is to seek advice from local experts who know about the shortcuts, and the pitfalls of surveys – and remember that surveys are costly!

APPENDIX. ADDRESSES OF INTEREST

1. UK Cochrane Collaboration,
   Summertown Pavillion,
   Middle Way,
   Oxford OX2 7LG

   Tel.: 01865 516300
   Fax: 01865 516311

   (For information on UK and worldwide Cochrane collaborations)

2. NHS Centre for Reviews and Dissemination,
   University of York,
   York YO1 5DD

   Tel.: 01904 433634
   Fax: 01904 433661

   (For information on systematic reviews of research)

3. NHS Executive,
   409 Wellington House,
   London SE1 8CG

   Tel.: 0171 972 4919
   Fax: 0171 972 4673

   (For information on Clinical Standards Advisory Group and Standing Medical Committee reports)

4. R&D Directorate,
   NHS Executive,
   GW52 Quarry House,
   Leeds LS2 7UE

   Tel.: 0113 2546194
   Fax: 0113 2546174

   (For information on the National Health Service Research and Development programme)

5. Wessex Institute of Public Health Medicine,
   Dawn House,
   Highcroft,
   Romsey Road,
   Winchester SO22 5DH

   Tel.: 01962 863511

   (For information on the National Health Service health technology assessment programme)

REFERENCES

Allan K 1994 Health data collection from general practice – a changing world. In: Richards B (ed). Conference proceedings – current perspectives in healthcare computing. BJHC Books, Weybridge, p 573

Davis P B, Yee R L, Millar J 1994 Accounting for medical variation: the case of prescribing activity in a New Zealand general practice sample. Social Science and Medicine 39: 367–374

De Grauw W J, van de Lisdonk E H, van den Hoogen H J, van Weel C 1995 Cardiovascular morbidity and mortality in type 2 diabetic patients: a 22 year historical cohort study in Dutch general practice. Diabetic Medicine 12: 117–122

Drever F 1994 Asthma, the changing scene? Population Trends 78: 44–46

Griffin E M, Vidgen G A, Hepworth J B 1994. Information use, information perceptions and information flows in primary care medical practice. Computer Methods and Programmes in Biomedicine 43: 207–211

Liverpool University 1995 Primary Care Data Project/Liverpool DISP III. Use of primary care data in commissioning. Departments of General Practice and Public Health, Liverpool University, Liverpool Sheffield Health Authority 1994

Lloyd D C, Harris C M, Clucas D W 1995 Low income scheme index: a new deprivation scale based on prescribing in general practice. British Medical Journal 310: 165–169

Majeed F A 1995 Deprivation payments to general practitioners. British Medical Journal 310: 1674

Majeed F A, Chaturvedi N, Reading R, Ben-Shlomo Y 1994a Monitoring and promoting equity in primary and secondary care. British Medical Journal 308: 1426–1429

Majeed F A, Cook D G, Anderson H R, Hilton S, Bunn S, Stones C 1994b Using patient and general practice characteristics to explain variations in cervical smear uptake rates. British Medical Journal 309: 476–477

Murphy P, Jenkins A 1995 MEDICS Project. Practice feedback report. Northumberland Health, Morpeth

Office of Population Censuses and Surveys 1995 The health of our children. Decennial supplement. HMSO, London

Pearson J, Barker J 1995 Developing a phased approach to needs assessment in primary care. Bromley Health, Bromley

Record M C, Spencer J A, Jones R H, Jones K P 1994 General practitioners' views about the statutory annual practice report. British Medical Journal 309: 849–852

Robson J, Falshaw M 1995 Audit of preventive activities in 16 inner London practices using a validated measure of patient population, the 'active patient' denominator. British Journal of General Practice 45: 463–466

Sheffield Health Authority 1994 LAPIS version 2. Locality and practice information system. User guide. Sheffield Health Authority, Sheffield

Sheldon T, Chalmers I 1994 The UK Cochrane Centre and the Centre for Reviews and Dissemination: respective roles within the information systems strategy of the NHS R&D Programme, coordination and principles underlying collaboration. Health Economics 3: 210–213

Somerset Health 1995 Continuous morbidity recording in general practice: The Somerset Project. Annual report. Somerset Health, Taunton

Somerset Health and Somerset Family Health Services Authority 1995 Somerset Morbidity Review 2(1). Public Health Analysis Unit, Somerset Health Commission, Taunton

Wennberg J, Gittlesohn A 1973 Small area variations in health care delivery. Science 182: 1102

Wilson A, McDonald P 1994 Comparison of patient questionnaire, medical record, and audio tape in assessment of health promotion in general practice consultations. British Medical Journal 309: 1483–1485

13

Using computer systems and new technology

Andrew Brooke

INTRODUCTION

Needs assessment is a complex issue, and general practitioners are increasingly being involved. It is not clear at present whether they will have an independent responsibility for this, but they will have a significant influence on needs assessment and health care provision whatever happens to locality commissioning and fundholding in future under different political scenarios.

Data collection (and analysis) for needs assessment is not dependent upon computer systems but has flourished with the spread of systems in primary care. Previously, analysis of information in the primary care setting depended on manually collected information in practice disease registers. This was useful at a practice level but inadequate for data collection at the suprapractice level. The urge for needs assessment in primary care is now mainly being driven by the necessity for health authorities and social services departments to purchase services and packages of care for people in their locality.

The role of computers in needs assessment lies partly in the gathering of morbidity and mortality data in general practice and also in its interpretation. In addition to practice-based clinical computer systems, there are also stand-alone systems which attempt to predict the needs of a population by simulating it.

CURRENT NHS COMPUTER STRATEGY

The National Health Service (NHS) Executive developed and published a national information management and technology strategy (Department of Health 1995). This strategy has the intention of improving the management and use of information within the NHS. The strategy includes the implementation of an information management and technology (IM&T) infrastructure. This infrastructure has several separate but complementary strands, which are all important in the gathering, transmission and analysis of data for needs assessment:

- Provision of a system of national standards for computer systems and for data handling
- Provision of physical connections between the different data providers and users in the NHS
- Improving the quality of information about patients and populations.

NHS COMMUNICATION NETWORK

An NHS communication network is currently being developed. This incorporates not only the transmission of data around the NHS but also voice and images, such as for telemedicine and radiology. It also has the potential for interactive access to libraries, bulletin boards and other sources of information such as waiting lists, poisons bureaux, etc. An initial service will be an NHS messaging system – a type of electronic mail. The system has the potential to transfer a patient's electronic record from his old to his new practice, or for referrals to be made electronically from the general practitioner to the consultant.

A major concern with such a national network is the security of the data and the necessity of complete confidentiality. A current problem is the issue of whether coding or encryption of the data is necessary prior to it being sent along the network. General practitioners are responsible for the safe custody of their patient's data and have considerable concerns about confidentiality given the apparent ease with which hackers gain access to databases in some other organizations.

GENERAL PRACTICE/DHA LINKS

The Links project is a scheme of local connections between individual general practices and their health authority DHA. It has the potential to act as a collecting system for data being provided by general practices to be collated by their DHA.

It commenced as an electronic system for the transmission of patient registration data, name, address, date of birth, etc. Its second phase involved the use of the system as a means for practices to make 'paperless' claims to their DHA for various services supplied to the patients for which a fee is due. The third phase involved transmission of data from hospital pathology laboratories direct to individual patient records on the general practice's computer.

NEW NHS NUMBERS

Part of the NHS information management strategy involves the replacement of the existing NHS number. This had been used in the past as a patient identifier. However, it developed in a rather haphazard way with a variety of differing number formats, which made it use-less as a means of uniquely identifying a patient electronically. The new NHS number scheme (which commenced with new numbers being allocated to infants born in December 1995) is expected to provide the necessary unique and unambiguous identifier to provide for accurate exchange of information between NHS health care systems. It consists of a 10-digit number, completely numeric, with the last digit a check number. The new NHS number contains no personal information.

COMPUTERS IN GENERAL PRACTICE

General practitioners have in recent years become greater users of computer systems in their practices, with over 85% of practices currently computerized. The types of system used range from single-user systems, now not so common, to the 'high-tech' practice networks with PCs on each desk. In between and accounting for the majority of systems are those with a single processor and many dumb terminals, frequently being used in consultations. Health visitors and district nurses also have access to computer systems. These are often a remote terminal used by several people connected by modem to the community health unit's computer. Hand-held systems are also used to gather data at source.

Data may be gathered by a single practice for its own use, for example age–sex data showing large numbers of young children registered with the practice, to support a bid for additional health visitor time. The practice might alternatively gather more clinical data; information on risk factors for ischaemic heart disease, or the prevalence of asthma within the practice to help decide the practice's priorities for primary or secondary disease prevention. Most practices have no difficulty identifying the need to introduce new clinical ideas into their practice. The main issue is to identify the priorities to allocate precious time to.

Health authorities also have a need to prioritize spending on different clinical issues. Their need is to gather data from a number of practices to provide reliable and accurate information to guide appropriate purchasing. They may choose to use a small number of representative practices for ease of coordination and communication. Alternatively, they may try to involve most or many local practices in the data gathering and sharing process as an educative and learning experience for the practices.

A crucial point here is to obtain agreement from the data collectors as to what should be collected and why. Clear protocols should be drawn up specifying the definition of the various conditions to be recorded. Otherwise, differences may appear between or even within practices that are purely due to inconsistent interpretation of a patient's symptoms and signs.

It is also important to specify the code to be used for a particular condition. For example, if 'deafness' is to be recorded, there are several quite different Read codes that might be used:

- 'Very deaf', Read code 2BL4 is derived from a set of codes to describe signs found on examination
- 'Conductive deafness', Read code F681, describes a specific diagnosis
- 'Deafness', Read code 1C13, is a symptom mentioned by the patient.

The person setting up a search for all deaf people either has to include the very wide range of codes that could possibly have been used. Or the searcher may assume that one particular code is the obvious one to search for, and may miss patients with alternative codes.

The use of a predefined template for data entry can avoid this problem.

To collate the data from a number of practices it must be feasible for the different systems used to extrude the data in a form that can be transferred to a central computer database. For relatively simple data analysis a spreadsheet or statistical program may suffice. These may be run within a practice using a PC. For more complex situations with many practices, with a wide range of conditions being analysed, a relational database may provide a more efficient way for data to be analysed. It is unlikely, however, that many practices would have the necessary skills to set this up themselves; most would need to liaise with their DHA to organize this.

Compatibility of the system with other users

Primary care computer systems evolved in a way that led initially to complete incompatibility between different general practice systems. Naturally there was no compatibility between any hospital system and a general practice computer. It became apparent that for data gathered over years to become useful it must be capable of being shared between clinicians, possibly also by academics and managers.

Several methods have been used to try and ensure compatibility of systems.

First, it is often helpful to have all the data coded in a similar way. In primary care most systems now use one or other version of Read coding. Other coding systems are also used, notably the International Classification of Diseases in hospital systems. Any approach towards system and data compatibility must tackle the problem of data being exchanged between coding systems. Read codes are likely to be the main coding system in NHS clinical information systems in the future.

A second and rather different way of moving towards system compatibility is the national system of accreditation of general practice computer systems. The philosophy here is to make any reimbursement of computing costs to general practitioners by FHSAs dependent on the relevant system having met the accreditation standards. The effect of this is likely to bring most systems up to an equivalent standard of functionality, but also to drive some smaller suppliers out of the primary care market and reduce the diversity that has always been a notable feature of general practice computing. Non-compatible systems may continue to develop but probably only in specialist niche markets.

As well as a system of accreditation there is also a national set of standards for data and all information technology products. Most major software suppliers have now had their normal clinical software accredited to the standard of the initial accreditation version 1. A new standard is introduced each year. Over a dozen suppliers have also had their fundholding software accredited. Up-to-date information on current accreditation status should be sought from the software supplier or a local DHA computer facilitator. The NHS Executive Information Management Group* can also supply up-to-date information.

Financial and resource implications of having a computer system

Computer systems are expensive in terms of their initial purchase and their maintenance, but also in terms of the costs of staff time to run the system. Most multi-user systems designed for the medium-to-large practice (47 partners) will cost up to £20 000 or £30 000. The ongoing annual software and hardware support fees and insurance for the system may amount to £2000–£4000 a year. The cost of staff time depends on the use made of the computer system by the practice and the quality of staff employed, but this may represent an annual cost of between £10 000 and £20 000.

The first general practice systems were purchased by enthusiastic general practitioners without any direct reimbursement, the cost coming directly out of their own pockets. It became apparent that to encourage the more widespread use of computers a form of partial reimbursement would be necessary. This was initially a scheme of reimbursement of up to 50% of the cost of system purchase and maintenance up to the limit of a budget applied by the DHA. The scheme has become a little more flexible since its inception, but for most practices the limit of reimbursement remains at 50%. A development of the computer reimbursement scheme came with the concept of fundholding in general practice. This took the form of a higher percentage reimbursement of computer-related costs. The costs of staff time and training remain a considerable expense for most practices. At a

*NHS Executive Information Management Group, IMG Information Point, c/o Cambridge and Huntingdon Health Commission, Primrose Lane, Huntingdon, Cambridgeshire PE18 6SE (Tel: 01480 415118).

time when many DHAs have had little room for increases in their reimbursement of staff costs to general practices, many practices have found that their use of computers is increasing. This uses up expensive staff time in addition to the practice's normal activities.

Despite the expense, the presence in a practice of a computer coordinator as a member of staff often helps to make much better use of the computer system. They can build up the expertise to assist other team members in the design of templates and the setting up of searches. They can also fulfil a valuable role in staff and doctor training, and in system security and data protection.

How to choose a system suitable for needs assessment

General practitioner systems were not initially designed for this purpose. Patient age–sex registers were an initial objective, followed by registration data. Then systems evolved to mimic the manual general practitioner record. Search and audit facilities followed, and now many systems look to supplant the manual record and improve the quality of the consultation.

When choosing a system a large user base is some indication of satisfaction with the system. A larger supplier may have more financial stability in the marketplace. It is important that your supplier is still in business or has not retired in 5 years' time.

The search and audit sections of the accredited systems are most likely to have desirable facilities, but it is wise to consult existing users of a system and the FHSA computer facilitator regarding the overall quality of the system.

The search and audit facilities on general practice computer systems still vary from extremely poor to barely adequate. Many systems still have little more than a facility to count numbers of entries of particular Read codes. Most systems will also be unable to do a search on any clinical data entered by the doctors as free uncoded text.

In some searches not all entries of a particular code may be required, only the most recent; the search facility should support this proviso. It should also be able to report numerical values such as blood pressure readings, or serum cholesterol levels.

It is important that the search facility can run complex searches with multiple operators such as 'and x, not y, if z'. It should also be able to run several searches simultaneously in a reasonable time and also without slowing the rest of the system down to a snail's pace.

Once the computer system has satisfactorily completed a search the data must be capable of being viewed on screen, printed out, or sent to a file either on floppy disk or electronically to another computer for more complex manipulation.

It is important that all or parts of the data can be printed in a very wide variety of user definable formats. For example, as a graph or a table, or just as a list of names. The practice might also want a variety of different age–sex bandings for reports produced for different purposes.

The practice might also want to print address labels from the results of the search, or a list of names with phone numbers for a receptionist to work through.

Part of the process of choosing a system must include the purchase cost, but also to be considered are the cost of maintenance, the quality of training provided and accessibility of system support – for example from the help desk in the event of urgent problems.

What if the present system is unsuitable?

If it proves inefficient to continue with an existing system then the painful prospect of a change of system must be considered. The reason for caution lies in the question of whether valuable data can be transferred intact and in a usable fashion to the new system.

If the existing system proves itself unsuitable, then a number of points must be considered before opting to change the system and supplier:

- Why is the system unsuitable?
- Is it possible to modify the software to make it easier to use or to provide the necessary functions?
- Would a hardware upgrade solve the problem?
- Would a new system fulfil all (or most) of the current needs and most envisaged future needs?
- Can data already gathered be readily transferred to the new system?
- Is a new system affordable?

Computer simulation for needs assessment

In addition to the use of computers in data gathering relating to real patients and its analysis, a relatively new role lies in computer simulation. The study of health care using computer simulation of clinical protocols, patients, clinicians and health care organizations and systems is a major new tool in health care management. It is useful in studying existing service delivery and is essential for studying if and how to provide any service for new clinical practice. The NHS is littered with policies introduced without adequate prior analysis.

If sufficient time and resources were available it would be possible to experiment in real life to understand how patient needs are best supplied. However, it would be invidious to contemplate this as a practical way of assessing needs in general practice. The issue is exceedingly complex, with horrendous ethical problems and, above all, would take too long to obtain any valid results.

Instead it is possible to use computer simulation (personal communication An Teallach Ltd) of clinical protocols to speed up knowledge acquisition of how a particular process behaves under different conditions.

There are several examples that illustrate the successful use of modelling and simulation for planning in non-health care situations. Architects draw up plans and build models, and increasingly these models are animated to give simulations. Designers of cars and aircraft build models that are animated in simulations to test aerodynamics, stress and customer appeal. It is now commonplace for pilots to train using a flight simulator and to use it to practice flying in various hypothetical situations – taking off, landing, night flying and engine failure for example. Virtual reality is beginning to be used in various ways to let people experiment with – or play in – new situations.

The common core of all these systems is a model which contains appropriate application knowledge. The structuring of this knowledge helps our understanding of many situations. If we can interact with the computer to change part of the model, then run a simulation and observe the consequences, we are in a position to explore the behaviour of the system that has been modelled. How much we can learn from the simulation depends on what we know already, how good the model is and what we can change.

The technological developments in computer systems that have made such simulations possible mean that we can use computer simulation to plan and manage health care. Until the development of powerful desk-top computers it was not possible to run a detailed simulation quickly enough to be useful for assessing health care needs and planning service delivery; but this can now be done.

It is important to recognize that the modelling and simulation of patient care described here is not an adaptation of systems for simulating manufacturing processes. People are not well modelled by single streams of sequential activities neatly separated by queues; they interact with the system being used. Simulation programs such as EpiPlan GP can be used with existing patient details from patient records or national or regional demographic data. Alternatively, it can use a simulated population with all the information relevant to the incidence and prevalence of any illness or illnesses including age, sex, economic status and socioeconomic factors such as housing or diet. Various scores and indicators can be incorporated to reflect attributes such as personality and education that will affect an individual's lifestyle and how he is likely to respond to health care screening or programmes such as disease prevention or fitness campaigns. An example of its use in managing a cervical screening programme is shown in Box 13.1.

Box 13.1 Using EpiPlan GP for cervical cytology needs assessment

Cervical cytology illustrates many aspects of the kind of problems that arise as general practitioners move from a reactive role to a proactive role in health care.

For a practice, the issues reside in managing the panel, and to be able to list and/or contact all potential patients and establish how many of those areas are at risk. Generally, a panel is dynamic and the extent of change will depend on the geographic area. At any one time there are:

- People who could be but are not registered (until they are ill)
- People who are registered but are elsewhere (but will not register elsewhere until they are ill)
- People who are temporary residents (either occasional or regular)
- People who are registered on the panel.

Even in semirural areas this inflow–outflow can be large, and its demographics are different for different conditions and can affect over 10% of the population. Younger people move for education and employment. For urban areas, mobility of 30–50% can be expected.

For the practice to improve the value of its cervical screening programme it will use EpiPlan models of:

1. The potential panel (so that it can explore levels and numbers at risk)
2. Attendances (same or new programme, campaigns and revised visit schedules)
3. Any opportunities to reorganize the service delivery (clinic times of day, reduced waiting times).

Then the simulations in EpiPlan will help answer the following questions:

- What is the likely rate of change and its impact on practice income?
- If the practice targeted those at greatest risk, how would it manage the increased workload?
- What numbers of tests/retests to purchase; who does the follow-up?
- Where to purchase (at the practice, community trust or special clinic)?
- Who will do what within the practice (responsibilities, records and reporting mechanisms)?

Also, the model and simulation will be used in team development – providing a non-threatening way to discuss the options in detail and to agree and plan any changes.

Help and advice

There are a number of fairly accessible sources of help for users struggling with their computer and needs assessment.

Local practices may have also tackled the same problem and come up with a solution. National and local user groups often represent a pool of considerable expertise in how to persuade your system to do what you would like it to do. User group bulletin boards are populated by experts who seem to spend all their time solving other people's problems.

Some DHAs have appointed local computer facilitators. Their role is often to advise and act to coordinate local users, but they can also help to assess computer systems and in some areas buy in training for practice staff. There was also the regional computer advisor who helped to coordinate regional policy. This rarely filters down as help to an individual practice. It remains to be seen with the demise of the region where the coordinating role will lie.

FUTURE DEVELOPMENT

The use of a PC and modem makes much medical and public health information directly available to the public. This may be by access to bulletin boards or by using e-mail or the Internet. It also facilitates direct communication of needs by the individual. The equipment for this may be in the home, but could also be available in public buildings, such as libraries, hospitals, or general practitioner surgeries. Vast amounts of information are available, but the problem is that there are no directories to guide the user immediately to the required information. A World Wide Web site (UK Med W3)* has been set up to improve access to medical information. This has links to other medical Web sites both in the UK and abroad.

The use of a PC in the consulting room opens up a large range of further options. By using a Windows-type interface a number of third party programs can be used during the consultation. CD-ROM can also be used to inform patients and aid in decision making.

A number of decision support programs have been developed for use in the consultation. There are programs currently in use to aid diagnosis in specific clinical areas such as dermatology, and also versions of electronic textbooks. These are not yet intended to replace a clinician in diagnosis and treatment, but to provide up-to-date information, in a readily accessible way. One such system is the clinical support system 'Mentor', developed by EMIS[†]. This is based on the *Oxford Handbooks of Medicine* and a dictionary containing over 20 000 key medical words or phrases. It can be used to provide information about a particular disease during the consultation for the benefit of either the doctor or the patient. The system can also be used to assist in the diagnostic process. The doctor will do this by entering a number of symptoms, signs or test results. The system then displays the best matches, divided up by both the importance of the disease suggested and by its prevalence. The system does not require a PC in the consulting room, and is regularly updated.

---

* http://www.ncl.ac.uk/~nphcare/GPUK/a_herd/topmenu.htm. World Wide Web site.

[†] Egton Medical Information Systems Ltd, Park House Mews, 77 Back Lane, Off Broadway, Horsforth, Leeds LS18 4RF (Tel: 0113 2591122).

An Teallach Ltd EpiPlan GP computer simulation program for needs assessment. Jane Bryon-Jones Cnoc Non Cnach by Catlodge, Laggon Bridge, Newbumore, RH20 1BT. Tel: 01528 544 312.

REFERENCES

Department of Health 1995 The impact on GP practices: implementing the infrastructure for information management & technology in the NHS. HMSO, London

14

The fluent artist

Andrew Harris

Probably only the proof-reader and editor turn to the last chapter, having read the whole book. Most readers will be looking for a synthesis of the many contributions, to help them understand not only what is current practice, but how it impacts on their work. It is with this intention that I approach the conclusion. It is clear that needs assessment means different things to different people. Becoming a competent practitioner requires fluency to interpret different 'languages'. I suggested that the working definition of needs assessment might be:

A systematic investigation into the health of some population, or group of people, sharing a common characteristic, in relation to existing public services, in order to meet a specific enquiry; and using methods which produce a sufficiently robust result, to be capable of influencing policy or practice, promoting the health of that group.

How has this stood up in the light of experience and practice in the field? It amply shows the purpose of needs assessment is to change policy or practice. It is integral to service planning. The necessity for a systematic approach has been emphasized by many authors. Even the simple approach of life cycle assessment outlined in Chapter 3 requires this. Judith Hooper, Nigel Edwards and Sarah Ann Ujah spell out in some detail the importance of planning, and offer a step-by-step guide. It means ad hoc needs assessments, without discovering what is already known and agreeing priorities and considering feasibility, are unadvisable. One of those steps is a practice diagnosis or health profile, and the authors stress that this alone is insufficient to constitute an assessment of need. It should be a systematic investigation of health. They warn that routine data tend to cause 'fishing trips', because it is available rather than because it is intrinsically useful. John Shanks and Sadru Kheraj demonstrate the potential of comparative needs assessments by aggregating and comparing standard data sets such as prescribing rates, practice demography and attendance at accident and emergency departments. However, they call for research to monitor the effectiveness of collecting and sharing such information, having been unable to discover a measure of its effectiveness. A report of the Somerset Morbidity project in Chapter 12 suggests that a valid assessment of morbidity may have impacted on district health authority contracting. There is generally an abundance of profiling with no clear end point or analysis to know if it is useful.

Needs assessment is a way of informing decision making, which otherwise might rely on crude routine data or lobby opinion. Chapter 2 highlights the danger of perpetrating inappropriate care, unless it is informed by evidence of need. To that we might add the danger of perpetrating care informed inappropriately by a poor measure of need. The routine data chapter reports that comparitive profiles of nursing staff led to collaborative work between general practice and community trusts. That is laudable, but insufficient. It is important that we develop routine data sets that reflect need and not just activity. It is clearly also necessary to bring together needs assessment project work and routine data, to enable a fuller picture to be seen by decision makers. Yvonne Doyle usefully asks three questions of those embarking on needs assessment, and these are equally applicable to those collecting information: What are we trying to achieve? Who are the main users? Who are the beneficiaries? A recurring theme throughout this book is achieving clarity about the precise information needed and its format (including getting the information technology right). That requires an understanding of available data sources and specific objectives (Chs 2 and 12). That is why there must be an aim to meet a specific enquiry in needs assessment. Having clear aims and objectives is advice that practitioners would be wise to heed, as the process becomes complex and spreads like ground elder, as data proliferates, rapidly obscuring its purpose.

That we are dealing with health is too often taken for granted. The opening chapter reminded us about the wide determinants of health, and the fact that health care was only a component of health-promoting activities. The theme is taken up by David Black and Pauline Craig, who demonstrate a plethora of health needs assessment projects which are not looking at health care. It appears that some of this healthy alliance and joint working has led to organizational restructuring and the establishment of resource centres. Changes in the practice of police and social workers, and provision of play areas and counselling advice, are other examples. Here there has been less emphasis on the technical methods used, and more on developing good working relations between different sectors, and between users and professionals. Chapters 2, 3 and 8 all stress the importance of good teamwork, and it must be recognized that the process of embarking on needs assessment is often a valuable team-building exercise. Changes in attitudes

and working practices may be hard to measure, but may be critical impacts of needs assessment activity that will have long-term benefits.

Needs assessment focuses on a population. Traditionally, general practice has regarded its main responsibility as the individual patient requesting care. Increasingly, interest has been shown in those registered with the practice, but not consulting, in part promoted by GP contract changes which remunerated immunization, surveillance and cervical screening activity. Community trusts have long been conscious of the safety net that they need to provide for the unregistered, homeless and highly mobile, work often led by the health visitor, one of the few practitioners explicitly trained in preventive care. In a primary care-led National Health Service, agreeing where responsibility lies for the full range of primary care, including prevention, is important. The opportunity to pilot new models of primary care outside the traditional GP contract, is one which crystallizes responsibilities for the population, and requires assessment of needs. Many general practices now recognize their crucial role in the community, but feel that they are ill equipped to look at the needs of the population, as they can barely cope with those consulting.

The opening chapter showed how demand has its own opportunity cost, and that meeting it does also. In other words, choosing to be solely reactive to demand, with the inherent time and resource allocations attributed to different patients, is implicitly choosing not to do something else. Needs assessment teaches us the importance of managing demand, and the mismatch between what we appear to want and what we need. Priorities change and are shaped by the process of needs assessment, and this learning exercise is a developmental gain from the process that should not be discounted. Containing the work of needs assessment and changing the clinical workload are possible by focusing on a smaller group sharing a common characteristic than the whole population. Much of the assessment may be integrated with day to day practice, but this does require prior planning. The opening chapter also explored the different meanings that writers have given the simple word 'need'. We learnt that needs are relative, and not fixed in time or place. We found that needs vary according to who judges them, and Jane Hopton and George Leahy emphasize how underlying values and principles affect those judgements, but are too often submerged in a debate about methods. Needs assessment can be used to deal with equity issues, but creating greater fairness requires agreement about whose values are to be used to assess equity. In public services there should be more explicit statements of value and principles which guide decision making. Need is about capacity to benefit: the definition is expressed in terms of its potential *impact* on health. Authors often found no measure of impact had been made, with interest focusing on findings, rather than the process by which those findings were translated into policy and practice. Thus we are often left with a judgement as to whether the assessment was sufficiently robust to influence, but due to other factors failed to do so, or whether it was insufficiently competent or powerful to exert influence.

When a doctor diagnoses an illness such as diabetes there are objective measures that can be used to confirm the competence of that assessment. But when he makes a diagnosis such as myalgic encephalomyelitis (ME), the correctness of that assessment is more open to debate. In this instance, we might ask how the diagnosis affected the management of the individual patient. Exactly so, primary care needs assessment: we cannot separate out with ease the complexities about how good is the design and conduct of the assessment from the crucial question about its impact on health. Indeed, because it is a proactive process, it is ethically behoven on its proponents to ensure that the process does have an impact. It needs to be timely, in a language appropriate to the policy maker or decision maker and answer the questions credibly in the context in which they were asked.

An academic author suggested that the needs assessment process was merely of heuristic value, that is useful for discovering knowledge, and promoting further enquiry, and, at least in relation to locality needs assessment, was not an appropriate means of achieving change. This is a timely caution, as interest grows in locality commissioning, but may be an unduly pessimistic view of the entire field of primary care needs assessment. Valerie Chisty and Christopher Heath report examples of an appointment of a therapist to a general practice, a new cryotherapy service and adoption of appropriate back pain management and referral guidelines. A leg ulcer clinic, a wider range of general practice family planning clinics, the creation of low-technology beds and the establishment of stroke clinics are examples of other impacts in Bromsgrove. Even in the localities chapter, the Salford project reported changes in contracts, extension of preventive care practice, such as promotion of exercise, and an impact on police activity. Community-oriented primary care reported in Chapter 11 led to a smoking abstension clinic, a mother and toddler group, and bereavement services. The Tower Hamlets Young Rehabilitation review in a community trust, reported in Chapter 9, resulted in changes in a consultant job, reconfigurations in therapy activity, a joint planning bid and a management-led project to implement chosen recommendations from the assessment.

The lesson that emerges from the reviewed fieldwork, and in particular the experience of evaluation reported in Chapter 2, is that there needs to be early and close collaboration between the researchers and implementors.

This often means cooperation between clinicians and management, throughout assessments to ensure it impacts on decision making. The reason that fundholders appear to have had some measure of success may be due to the fact that the researcher and implementor may be the same person, or at any rate in direct-line management. Working across organizations and between cultures has always been more difficult. The limited impact of needs assessment may be more a reflection of the imperfections in corporate management, and lack of clarity about individual needs of stakeholders at the outset. It was suggested in Chapter 1 that common organizational pathologies may be eased by needs assessment. It may help distinguish vested interests from priority needs, focus on the detailed practical steps rather than macro policy, and at the same time ensure that opportunities beyond the confines of the contracting process for an impact on population health are considered.

This is why the chapter by Laurann Yen and Liz Haggard is so important, where managerial views are used to explore the role of community trusts. Needs assessment was found to meet a corporate need, reconciling the strategic and operational, monitoring preventive care programmes and influencing purchasing. Identification of inappropriate patterns of care, promoting good practice, and helping look at new models of care are all described. Here management is creating an environment in which professional practice is valued and given time to reflect on shared information. Thus we may legitimately see needs assessment as creating a working environment which is better equipped to promote health, and this may well be an essential early phase in developing its effectiveness.

Rapid appraisal techniques, reported by Scott Murray and Steve Gillam, show impacts such as the establishment of dog free zones, new bus routes and provision of toys in the waiting area. An important aspect of such work is that it is an effective way of involving users, and facilitates change as it goes along. This may make evaluation of its impact more difficult, but its developmental potential in the long run is promising, if it engages key stakeholders across professional, managerial and consumer groups.

The complex language of needs assessment not only requires mutual understanding of what we mean by the words we use, but also a deeper understanding about each other's work culture and priorities. A needs assessment performed within a hierarchical professionally led person culture will be difficult to implement in a corporate top management-led culture, and vice versa. To be a practitioner of needs assessment, not only are technical scientific skills necessary to ensure the methods are valid and robust but sophisticated skills from the realms of art and the humanities are needed. It is suggested that the failure to synthesize assessments in different cultures –

particularly biomedical and sociological, has been a brake on the potential impact of needs assessment.

An example of the combination of creativity and scientific validity are some of the techniques described by the Gabbays in their fascinating chapter on the needs of hard-to-reach groups. The projects described show how people have built on other's work, and used initiative and intelligence to collect information by often unorthodox ways to paint the picture of small groups with particular needs. Perhaps the most scientifically valid technique is that described as epidemiologically based needs assessment. The key is the triangulation of effectiveness information, population data and service information. Andrew Stevens and Mike Sadler point out how critical it is to ensure that the size of the population is suitable for the approach, and to be sure that something can be done, before embarking on this resource intensive exercise.

The importance of triangulation is crucial when less well defined techniques such as community health projects are used. Too often there has been inadequate triangulation, with considerable loss of validity. This inevitably reduces the robustness of the findings, and makes them less likely to effect policy or practice. Choosing valid tools, or creating valid methods, and implementing them in a way that enables them to be reliably repeated, are basic requirements emphasized in several chapters. There is no 'off the peg' primary care needs assessment tool, nor should there be. Each assessment has to be built up in a creative way, to suit its purpose and locality. There is much information in this book to guide people in that task. The real challenge is to preserve some scientific credibility whilst building into the process the means of implementation and influence of the findings. This will require a mix of skills and cultures, and early and ongoing collaboration with other people and different organizations.

The fluent practitioner should view his task as a combination of that of an interpreter with that of an artist. The interpreter listens not just to the words, but to the whole sentence, and pays attention to tone, emphasis and body language in assessing meaning. The most important skill learnt by an art student is to learn how to see, when they look, and realize the colours, depths, shapes, objects they had not seen before. Just so the assessor of need who must sensitively recognize the different measures of need, their different characteristics and values. The next stage is creative. The interpreter synthesizes what he has learnt, and translates the meaning into the appropriate language. The artist chooses his colours, shape and tone to paint a picture with the meaning and feeling he wishes to create. Just so the needs assessor, who must be a fluent artist, building up pictures and descriptions into true stories, that have a lasting impact on their readers. It is the most creative challenge in today's health service.

Index

Alphabetical arrangement is word-by-word.
Added to the page number, f denotes a figure,
t denotes a table.

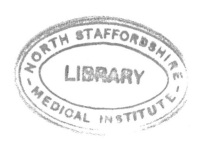